ROUTLEDGE LIBRARY EDITIONS: NURSE EDUCATION AND NURSING CARE

Volume 1

COMMUNITY NURSING

COMMUNITY NURSING

Research and Recent Developments

G. BAKER, J. M. BEVAN,
L. McDONNELL
AND
B. WALL

Routledge
Taylor & Francis Group

LONDON AND NEW YORK

First published in 1987 by Croom Helm Ltd.

This edition first published in 2026
by Routledge
4 Park Square, Milton Park, Abingdon, Oxon OX14 4RN

and by Routledge
605 Third Avenue, New York, NY 10158

Routledge is an imprint of the Taylor & Francis Group, an informa business

British Library Cataloguing in Publication Data
A catalogue record for this book is available from the British Library

ISBN: 978-1-041-11658-5 (Set)
ISBN: 978-1-041-11088-0 (Volume 1) (hbk)
ISBN: 978-1-041-11099-6 (Volume 1) (pbk)
ISBN: 978-1-003-65826-9 (Volume 1) (ebk)

DOI: 10.4324/9781003658269

Publisher's Note
The publisher has gone to great lengths to ensure the quality of this reprint but points out that some imperfections in the original copies may be apparent.

Disclaimer
The publisher has made every effort to trace copyright holders and would welcome correspondence from those they have been unable to trace.

Community Nursing
Research and Recent Developments

G. BAKER, J.M. BEVAN, L. McDONNELL and B. WALL

CROOM HELM
London • New York • Sydney

Croom Helm Ltd, Provident House, Burrell Row,
Beckenham, Kent, BR3 1AT
Croom Helm Australia, 44-50 Waterloo Road,
North Ryde, 2113, New South Wales

Published in the USA by
Croom Helm
in association with Methuen, Inc.
29 West 35th Street
New York, NY 10001

British Library Cataloguing in Publication Data

Community nursing: research and recent
    developments.
    1. Community health nursing — Great Britain
    — History — 20th century
    I. Baker, G.
    610.73'43'0941   RT98
    ISBN 0-7099-4415-2

Library of Congress Cataloging-in-Publication Data

ISBN 0-7099-4415-2

Printed and bound in Great Britain by Mackays of Chatham Ltd, Kent

CONTENTS

Contents

Contents

Contents

Contents

Contents

PREFACE AND ACKNOWLEDGEMENTS

This book arose out of a project commissioned by the Department of Health and Social Security (see page 11) and so we must first record our thanks for the grant provided by the Department over the period 1980 to 1984. We are most grateful to Dr Doreen Rothman, OBE, DHSS Liaison Officer to the Health Services Research Unit of the University of Kent for her support and assistance throughout the period of the project and to the present.
Professor Michael Warren, first Director of the Health Services Research Unit (1971-1984) by example and advice taught us much about the nature of Health Service Research and what to aim for in terms of quality and applicability. We owe a great debt of gratitude to him for this and for the specific help and guidance he gave us with the project on which this book is based. We must also record our warm thanks to the present Director of the Health Services Research Unit, Professor Louis Opit for allowing us the use of the facilities of the Unit to complete this book.
When the Department of Health and Social Security commissioned us to undertake this work, they put before us as a model the approach adopted by Donald Hicks in 'Primary Health Care: A Review' (published in 1976 by HMSO). Though we never met him we learned a great deal from his review and were saddened to learn of his death as we were in the course of writing this book. One characteristic we have in common with him and should mention is that we are all in a sense writing as 'outsiders' in that none of us have either nursing or medical qualifications. This has the drawback that we may lack an understanding of what it is to work in this field but it did at least mean that we approached our task without any preconceptions arising

from being a member of any of the professions whose innovative activities we were exploring - though no doubt we have our own prejudices and hope they have not intruded too much.

At this point we should mention a convention we have adopted. This is that following fairly general usage in the nursing press, we have generally used 'she' or 'her' etc. when referring to nurses. When referring to medical practitioners or others, we have tried to remain neutral as to whether that person was male or female - except of course where we have quoted directly from a publication.

Because we were 'outsiders' we had to rely particularly on the generosity of those whose help we sought in discovering what was going on in community nursing and our deepest thanks go to those we mention below for all the help they gave us.

At an early stage in the project we approached those bodies (as they then were) most directly concerned with our field of interest with requests for help to which they very generously responded. The bodies were:-

The Council for the Training and Education of Health Visitors (now superseded with the coming into being of the United Kingdom Central Council for Nursing, Midwifery and Health Visiting);
The General Medical Services Committee, British Medical Association;
The Health Visitors' Association;
The Panel of Assessors for District Nurse Training (now superseded following the coming into being of the United Kingdom Central Council for Nursing, Midwifery and Health Visiting);
The Queen's Nursing Institute;
The Royal College of General Practitioners;
The Royal College of Nursing.

The individuals representing these bodies, together with a number of others approached individually, who were all so helpful, we list below and thank them all very much for the time and trouble they took in providing us with the information and comment we needed. They were:-

Eunice Buggey, Dr Keith Bolden, June Clark, Baroness Caroline Cox of Queensberry, Dr Peter Enoch, Ainna Fawcett-Henesy, Audrey Grey, Dr Lisbeth Hockey, OBE, Marion Holloway, Dr Peter Kielty, Dorcas Knowles, Dr Charlotte Kratz, Dr Barrie

Preface and Acknowledgements

Reedie, Barbara Robottom, Dr Brian Salter, Barbara Stilwell, Margaret Thwaites, Jenny Triptree, Dr Alison While, Geraldine White, Margaret White, Margot White, Susan Willis, Dr Jennifer Wilson-Barnett, and Joyce Wiseman.

We are also most grateful for all the Nursing Officers in Districts who responded to our ques-tionnaires especially at a time when they were pre-occupied with the problems of the 1982 restructur-ing of the National Health Service.

Our warmest thanks too are due to the Librar-ians who assisted us giving generously of their time. In particular:-

Sue Cover, Librarian, Kent Postgraduate Medical Centre, Canterbury;
Helga Perry, formerly Librarian, Nurse Education Centre, Canterbury and Thanet Health District;
David Rumsey, District Librarian, William Harvey Hospital, Ashford;
John Jefferies, formerly Assistant Librarian, University of Kent at Canterbury (who organized our Medline search).

We also thank the Librarian at the Royal Society of Health, Kate Jones, and staff of the Library of the Royal College of Nursing, for their help in providing material.

No list of thanks would be complete without reference to our friend and colleague Associate Professor Kozo Tatara of the University of Osaka Medical School, Japan whose perceptive and sym-pathetic studies of community nursing in this country opened our eyes to many developments and possibilities in this field.

Finally we offer our thanks to all those who have thought up and written about innovations in community nursing, those who have tried them out in practice and those who have carried out studies of such innovations. Without their efforts there would have been no point to this book.

With all this help we are conscious of the responsibility that we have had to produce some-thing worthwhile - needless to say any short com-ings, errors and omissions are ours alone.

Gail Baker, John Bevan, Linda McDonnell and Barbara Wall

Our report to the Department of Health Social Sec-urity on the original project was in four parts as follows -

Preface and Acknowledgements

HSRU Report No. 46, Developments in Community Nursing Within Primary Health Care Teams

Part I   -   General review and summary
Part II   -   A review of the literature 1974-82
Part III -   Report of the survey addressed to Chief Nursing Officers
Part IV   -   Report on consultations held with representatives of professional bodies and other selected members of the nursing and medical professions and discussion of the research priorities arising from the project

Although these reports are now out of print, copies are held at the Library of the University of Kent at Canterbury and may be consulted, if desired, on application to the Library.

Chapter One

INTRODUCTION

WHAT THIS BOOK IS AND IS NOT ABOUT

Titles of books are inevitably short and beg
as many questions as they answer. This one is no
exception.
So whom do we mean by 'community nurses'? We
have confined our attention to those most closely
involved in the day-to-day work of providing primary health care (that is, health care outside hospitals or the hospital services). In fact we have
taken this to mean district nurses, health visitors
(excluding, however,their work in the school health
service), health authority employed treatment room
nurses and practice employed nurses. We will
explain below more precisely who these generally
are. Also included are those with lesser or no
formal nursing qualifications working in teams led
by one of the above types of community nurses.
This means that we are excluding some who have a
claim for inclusion in the collective 'community
nursing'; for example, community psychiatric nurses
and community midwives are not included, nor shall
we consider those involved in school health services only. Even so, as will become evident, the
range of nursing activities and nursing specialisms
falling within the terms of reference we have set
ourselves is quite wide.
Having defined what we mean by community nursing, we turn next to the phrase 'recent developments' in the title. By 'recent' we mean those
documented since 1974 - though in order to set
these in context we shall have to look further back
(see Chapter Two). By 'developments' we refer to
innovations in role and activities. These will
include changes in clientele served, developments
of specialist functions such as 'stoma adviser',

1

Introduction

hospital community liaison functions, issues relating to the degree of autonomy of community nurses
in relation to medical or other caring professions,
including the administrative and managerial relationships of community nurses to other 'carers'. We
shall be concerned to document both the developments actually tried out and ideas about future
innovations aired in medical and nursing circles
which looked promising, even if not (as far as is
known) actually tried out in practice.
    This brings us to the word 'research' in the
title. We are concerned here with evaluative research undertaken in relation to developments in
community nursing. What sort of evidence was used
by writers in recommending the adoption of new
developments, or for that matter to discourage
their spread through the health services? Is the
approach to the gathering of evidence scientific
and practical in orientation? Would the conclusions drawn be accepted by any reasonable person
and, even if they were, would they matter in
practical terms?
    Finally this leaves us with the question, is
there any research needed into developments (existing and potential)? We shall spend some time pre-
senting views on this from a number of medical and
nursing professional organizations and professions
as well as ourselves.
    Now that we have described, in broad outline,
what this book is about, the remainder of this
chapter will be devoted to some fuller explanations
about the types of community nurses with which we
shall be concerned, the origin of the investigation
on which this book is based, and the sources of
information used.

SOME EXPLANATIONS

Health visitors, district nurses, treatment room
nurses, practice nurses and the National Health
Service
        The Department of Health and Social Security
in a memorandum in 1977 (CNO(77)8 - the appendix)
described the categories of community nurses with
which this book is concerned as follows:

        The Health Visitor is a family visitor
    and an expert in child health care. She is
    trained to understand relationships within the
    family and the effects upon these relation-
    ships of the normal processes of growth and

ageing and events such as marriages, births and deaths. She is concerned with the promotion of health and the prevention of ill health through giving education, advice and support, and by referring to the general practitioner or to other National Health Service or statutory or voluntary services where special help is needed. The health visitor is a professional in her own right, and she initiates action on behalf of her clients and refers to other agencies as she considers appropriate. She makes a very special contribution by visiting families who may have no other regular contact with health services, or who may be visited by no other voluntary or statutory worker, so that she alone may be in a position to identify physical, mental or social illness or family breakdown, and to alert others as appropriate. She is the leader of a team which may include SRNs, SENs and nursing auxiliaries working in schools or clinics. The scope for the employment of supporting staff, and the nature of the tasks which the health visitor delegates to them, will vary according to the needs of the population she serves.

The District Nurse is a SRN who has received post basic training in order to enable her to give skilled nursing care to all persons living in the community including in residential homes. She is the leader of the district nursing team within the primary health care services. Working with her may be SRNs, SENs and nursing auxiliaries. It is the district nurse who is professionally accountable for assessing and re-assessing the needs of the patient and family, and for monitoring the quality of care. It is her responsibility to ensure that help, including financial and social, is made available as appropriate. The district nurse delegates tasks as appropriate to SENs, who can thus have their own caseload, but who remain wholly accountable to the district nurse for the care that they give to patients. The district nurse is accountable for the work undertaken by nursing auxiliaries who carry out such tasks as bathing, dressing frail ambulant patients, and helping other members of the team with patient care.

Treatment room nurses are employed by some (Area) Health Authorities. These nurses

3

undertake a wide variety of treatments in health centres or general practice premises. In other (Area) Health Authorities the district nursing team undertake these tasks as well as their domiciliary work.

Some general practitioners employ nurses on nursing and/or reception duties, and these are known as practice nurses. They may work alongside (Area) Health Authority employed nurses who are attached to the practice, but seldom undertake work outside the surgery premises. They may be included in training programmes organised by the (Area) Health Authority.

To practise as a health visitor, a person must have a minimum of five 'O' levels, be a registered general nurse and have approved obstetric training and experience (that is either she must possess the full midwifery qualification or have taken a specially organized twelve week obstetric nursing course) and have completed further training leading to the award of the health visitor's certificate. (This involves a training period of one calendar year, roughly equally divided between theory and practice, followed by a minimum of nine weeks supervised practice. It is also possible for a person with the appropriate academic qualifications to take a degree course which allows for health visiting studies within a composite programme of education and training for the general register, and some centres organize special courses for those already possessing a degree.)

The syllabus for the health visitor's certificate embraces the development of the individual, the individual in the group, development of social policy, social aspects of health and disease, and the principles of, and practice of, health visiting. The present requirements necessary to practise as a health visitor date essentially from the National Health Service (qualification of health visitors) regulations, 1964 (para.2a) which made provision for the certificate of the Council for the Education and Training of Health Visitors (CETHV), the then statutory body responsible for health visitor training - whose function has now been subsumed within the UKCC framework (see page 41) 'to become a condition for employment to practise as a health visitor in the United Kingdom' (Owen, 1983). However, training requirements along broadly similar lines have existed on a national

Introduction

basis since 1925. Prior to this it was not required that a health visitor be a trained nurse or midwife; so a university degree would suffice as a
precondition for entering upon specific health
visiting training.
The definition of the role of the health
visitor given earlier makes it clear that it is a
very wide one. In the past the role has been even
wider. For instance, the implementation of the
Local Authority Social Services Act (1970) led to
the transfer 'to Local Authority Social Services
Departments of responsibility for the home help
service of which some health visitors had been
pioneer organizers, and for the day-care of pre-
school children for which health visitors had long
accepted full responsibility' (Health Visitors'
Association, 1981). Moreover the health visitor, as
the description on page 2 states, is a professional
in her own right having a statutory duty in relation to attending upon homes and families of recently born children; and having freedom, particularly in the care of young children, within the
policy guidelines of her employing authority, to
initiate contact and determine their subsequent
frequency independently from the general practitioner. This independence from the general practitioner in terms of decision making within certain
spheres of her activity is a distinctive feature of
the health visitor as compared with the other types
of community nurse we shall be considering.
As from September 1981 those seeking to enter
the practice of district nursing must satisfy
requirements somewhat akin to those for health
visitors. Thus they must be a registered general
nurse, usually having five or more 'O' levels,
having a minimum of one year's post-registration
experience and having followed training leading to
the award of the national certificate in district
nursing. The minimum training requirements for
this qualification are nine months study, the first
six months of which is approximately two-thirds
theory, one-third practical, followed by three
months of supervised practice. The syllabus for
the theoretical aspect of the course includes
sections on the theories and principles of district
nursing, trends in medical practice, social sci-
ences and social administration. In some educational institutions part of the district nurses'
training is given in the form of lectures common
also to those working for the health visitor's
certificate.

5

Introduction

Prior to 1981 it was possible to be a district nurse without having to obtain the national certificate in district nursing though that certificate was available and generally encouraged. In fact, it appears (DHSS, 1981) that most of those practising as full district nurses (as distinct from those helping them) had received district nursing training (about 80% were thus qualified). The same publication reveals that a substantial proportion of state enrolled nurses assisting district nurses had also obtained some district nursing training.

The role of the district nurse is much more self-evidently located within the heartland of general nursing than that of the health visitor, though the district nurse particularly when working in her patients' homes must obviously practise in relative isolation from other medical and nursing support compared with her colleagues in a hospital situation.

Originally the district nurse and health visitor provided care in patients' homes only but (see page 20) since 1968 it has been possible to attend patients also in surgery or clinic premises. The health authority employed treatment room nurse, and the practice employed nurse (who also usually tends to work in a treatment room or at least in the surgery premises of a general practitioner) do not have to obtain at present any qualifications other than those necessary for them to undertake the nursing activities which constitute their work - they are thus usually registered general or state enrolled nurses. Recently a steering group representative of nursing and medical organizations agreed to recommend a course of training for practice nurses (see page 93).

All but the last of these nurses (i.e. the practice employed nurse) are direct employees of the National Health Service and form part of the total nursing services of a district health authority. We should explain that in England (and the position, questions of scale apart, is broadly similar in Wales and Scotland), the National Health Service is administered according to the following scheme. England is divided into 14 health regions and (since 1982) each of these is divided into a number of district health authorities, amounting in all to 192 district health authorities in England, each serving populations ranging from less than 100,000 in one district to over 800,000 in the case of the most populous district. The district health authority is divided into units of management which

may for example be a large hospital, a collection
of hospitals, a community unit comprising the staff
and facilities involved in the provision of community services of the district health authority, or
units responsible for providing care to particular
care groups, such as the elderly or the very young,
or mental illness services. Where there is a community unit, the community nursing services of a
district health authority will usually all be provided by this unit. Where units are associated
with special care groups, community nurses may be
administered by different units, according to their
function. For example, health visitors may belong
to the unit with a remit to provide among other
services maternity care and care for the very
young, district nurses to the unit for the care of
the elderly. (By community we generally mean those
services not provided through the main acute, psychiatric and other specialized hospitals of the
district.)

The 1974 reorganization of the National Health
Service had the effect of arranging the management
of all nursing within a district* in a hierarchy
with the district nursing officer (or chief nursing
officer as he/she sometimes subsequently came to be
called) at the peak of the pyramid.

The nursing manpower of the district was
divided into divisions, for example the acute division, psychiatric division, community division,
each headed by a divisional nursing officer directly accountable to the district nursing officer.
Within the community division, where it existed,
there was a hierarchy of senior nursing officers
and nursing officers leading down to the health
visitors and district nurses who actually provided
the bulk of the face-to-face care for clients and
patients with the help of less fully trained staff
working under their direction. When units of management covering between them all aspects of the
patients' services provided by a district were set
up following the 1982 restructuring of the National
Health Service, the idea was initially that they
would be managed by a trio comprising an administrator, a director of nursing services and a representative medical practitioner (i.e. a consultant
or possibly a general practitioner).

---

*There were not at that time district health
authorities, but districts as geographical entities
in roughly their present form came into being at
that point - see Levitt and Wall, 1984.

Introduction

The hierarchical management structure of a
unit for nurses, from the director of nursing services downwards remained essentially similar to
that of the superseded divisions. However, since
the trio managing the unit were to be collectively
responsible to the district health authority for
the functioning of the unit, this implied that the
chief nursing officer of the district would no
longer be regarded as the hierarchical superior of
the unit's director of nursing services.

In any event, at the time of writing a further
change in the management of units is taking place
in that general managers of units are being appointed who will have sole responsibility for the
management of their respective units. The implication of this is that nursing staff in a unit will
in a general sense be accountable to the unit general manager via the director of nursing services
(or whatever the senior nurse in the unit is termed
in a particular unit.)

At district and regional level, general managers are now also largely in post and although
there will still be a designated senior nurse responsible for professional nursing matters, the post
of chief nursing officer of a district need not,
and frequently does not, exist. The position is
far from clear as district general managers formulate plans of management structures within their
districts but it does look as though there may, and
probably will, be a lot more variation in this respect from district to district than has been the
case since 1974. Moreover, in the case of community nursing services, further uncertainty exists
as amongst other things the report by the Community
Nursing Review Team (see page 101) appointed by the
government has made recommendations concerning
changes in the organization of the service. It
does now seem unlikely that family practitioner
committees will take over the responsibility for
community nursing (see page 30).

Within the National Health Service, general
medical services are provided by a very different
arrangement. They are provided in particular by
general medical practitioners (GPs or family doctors) who are in contract to provide such services
with family practitioner committees which are organizationally separate from the health authorities
at regional level and below, and at present the
boundaries of areas covered by family practitioner
committees do not coincide as a rule with those of
just one district health authority. In principle

Introduction

the general practitioner contracts as an independent entrepreneur to provide general medical services and a central feature of the general medical services in the United Kingdom is that members of the public are, as far as is practical, free to choose which GP they should be registered with and vice versa. This means that the collection of patients who are registered with a practice are scattered over an area served also by often a number of other general practitioners.

As an independent contractor, the general practitioner provides premises from which to discharge his or her obligations, within broad limits as he/she judges appropriate, and employs staff to assist in the work of the practice such as secretaries and receptionists and sometimes practice employed nurses. These staff are employees of the general practitioner(s), an individual if practising single-handed, or more commonly of a group or partnership of general practitioners who share facilities and staff, and it is to the GP or the partnership alone that they are accountable.* Thus in particular the practice employed nurse is directly accountable to the employing general practitioner (or group of general practitioners) unlike the remainder of the community nurses as we have defined them (see page 1) who are health authority employed and are not accountable directly to a member of the medical profession. However, health authority employed community nurses, and in particular district nurses and health visitors, may be attached to general practitioners, so that the patients for which the community nurses in question are responsible are those of the general practitioner(s) to whom they are attached (rather than those defined as being within a particular geographical area or patch - which also still happens, and was common 25 years or more ago). Moreover, the general practitioner refers, especially to the district nurse, patients who actually require nursing care outside hospital. Whether or not a district nurse is attached to a practice, most of her clientele originate from the general practitioner. With the health visitor it is different, she is more independent of the general practitioner in

---

*Though sometimes where GPs work from health authority owned premises such as health centres, the ancillary staff working for the GP are employed by the health authority for convenience of administration.

the choice and management of care of her clientele,
especially among her primary client group, the very
young and their mothers; but especially in the case
of the elderly there is a need to liaise with general practitioners and other members of the primary
health care team. (The primary health care team
essentially comprises the general practitioner and
community nurses, particularly if they are in an
attachment scheme.)
     One final fact about the provision of care
that should be mentioned is the crucial central
position of the general practitioner in the provision of health care within the National Health
Service. It is only with the general practitioner
that a member of the general public has a direct
contractual relationship. It is to the general
practitioner that patients must go if they require
not only general medical care but if they need services on an outpatient or inpatient basis of the
hospital (except in an emergency) and indeed the
general practitioner is often the initial point of
contact when one needs district nursing services or
treatment-room care. Because the general practitioner is the only person within the National
Health Service who has a continuing responsibility
for named patients, as long as they are registered
with him or her, the GP is the only person who has
the opportunity (though not any obligation to
record particular details) to maintain a continuing
record of care provided by the National Health
Service to that person.

Why we have concentrated on the last decade
     Basically there are two reasons. First, the
National Health Service underwent a quite radical
reorganization with effect from 1st April, 1974
which in particular involved the bringing together
of hospital and community nurses (apart from practice employed nurses) under the same authority.
(Previously community nurses had been part of the
Health Department of Local Authorities.) Secondly,
the Department of Health and Social Security, who
commissioned the study on which this book is based,
had previously commissioned, and the HMSO had published, a major work, Primary Health Care (Hicks,
1976) which covered among other things developments
in community nursing up to about 1974.
     It is of course impossible to understand what
happened from 1974 onwards without some knowledge
of relevant events before then - but we have concentrated our literature search for developments in

community nursing from 1974 and asked those we questioned to report developments and ideas arising from, roughly speaking, the same point.

How this work arose

The brief, agreed with the DHSS when the project on which this book is based was commissioned, was as follows:

The purpose of the proposed project is to identify, describe and assess, schemes involving developments in community nursing services including in particular new approaches to cooperation between general practitioners and nurses in the provision of primary health care. The emphasis would be on schemes arising since 1974 or not already covered in existing reviews such as 'Primary Health Care: A Review' by Donald Hicks (1976) and would aim to cover all schemes within the above terms of reference, not only published work or those which were (or are) the subject of some research investigation.... The primary objective of the study would be to provide information to the DHSS which would be of assistance in formulating a long term strategy for research and development in primary health care. It would also of course have obvious applications in disseminating information about developments in aspects of primary health care covered within the National Health Service and to research organizations. The project would generally be confined to the United Kingdom and mainly to schemes and studies in England.*

Reports in relation to the above purposes have been presented to the DHSS and this book represents an up-dated version of the main material presented in these reports.

Sources of information on which this work is based

1. The literature review. Several methods were used to try to obtain a comprehensive survey of the literature from the beginning of 1974 until the end of 1984 (though we have included some work published since where this seemed particularly important).

*In the event the last restriction was not observed, at least in the literature search.

Introduction

The following journals and magazines were searched issue by issue from the beginning of 1974:

British Medical Journal
Community Development Journal
Family Practitioner Services Journal
General Practitioner
Health and Social Services Journal
Health Bulletin
Health Visitor
Lancet
Journal of Advanced Nursing
Journal of Community Nursing (now Journal of District Nursing)
Journal of Epidemiology and Community Health (formerly British Journal of Preventive and Social Medicine)
Journal of the Royal College of General Practitioners
Midwife, Health Visitor and Community Nurse
Midwives Chronicle
Nursing
Nursing Focus
Nursing Mirror)
Nursing Times)   now combined
Public Health
Pulse
The Practitioner
Practice Team
Royal Society of Health Journal
Update

Lists of current literature were searched from 1981 onwards, including Nursing Research Abstracts, Health Services, and General Medical Practice (which are all produced by the DHSS), the Royal College of Nursing Bibliography, and the King's Fund list of additions to the library.

Articles obtained in the above searches, and books and pamphlets acquired for the project have been in turn searched for any references they gave. This 'trawl' produced relevant items not found in earlier searches.

A search using 'Medline' was made and yielded a number of relevant items but only a few were not already in our lists, and these were mainly in foreign journals.

Representatives of professional organizations who were consulted in connection with the project made suggestions about items to include.

Introduction

In addition to this primary literature search, key documents relating to the subject from before 1974 were consulted, though not directly reviewed.

2. The survey addressed to chief nursing officers of health authorities in England. A postal survey was addressed to 194 chief nursing officers of all district health authorities in England. 74% responded with information, 9% had no schemes or views to put forward and 17% refused or did not respond. The survey was made in mid 1982 with a further approach to responding authorities for updating on the schemes in early 1983. The survey was concerned with identifying: developments already in operation either in the district of the respondent or elsewhere which the respondent thought ought to be brought to our attention; suggestions for developments in community nursing made by respondents and suggestions for research in community nursing (with a distinction being made between research which was needed generally and research which should be given priority).

3. Consultations held with representatives of professional bodies and other selected members of the nursing and medical professions, including in particular discussions of research priorities arising from the project at the time of these consultations (based mainly on information obtained from sources 1 and 2 above).

Interviews were held with representatives of professional organizations in nursing and medicine (listed below) during the period December 1982 to May 1983 as well as with other members of the profession known to have an active interest in the subject of the project. Representatives of the following bodies were interviewed:

Council for the Education and Training of Health Visitors*
General Medical Services Committee, British Medical Association
Health Visitors' Association
Panel of Assessors for District Nurse Training*
Queen's Nursing Institute
Royal College of General Practitioners
Royal College of Nursing

*Subsequently the functions of these were taken over by the appropriate parts of the framework of the United Kingdom Central Council for Nurses.

Introduction

4. Information about on-going research. From various sources, including those listed above, but in addition lists of research ongoing, research projects in progress that appeared to be within our terms of reference were identified and followed up to obtain a report on progress and findings when available.

Chapter Two

THE CONTEXT IN WHICH DEVELOPMENTS IN COMMUNITY
NURSING HAVE TAKEN PLACE SINCE 1974

INTRODUCTION

Developments in community nursing, as in any
other sphere of activity, do not take place in a
vacuum. They are a response to, or at least influenced by, a number of factors. Some of these
factors were evident long before the start of the
period with which we are chiefly concerned, but
still have an important influence on events; some
emerged at the start of our period and are in
effect one reason for choosing this starting point;
some have manifested themselves since 1974.

In this chapter, we consider factors, issues
and influences and in the following chapter turn to
specific documents such as circulars and reports of
the DHSS, professional organizations and the like.

NUMBERS (whole time equivalents) OF COMMUNITY
NURSES AND INFORMATION ON THEIR WORKLOAD - AND
INFORMATION ON THE NUMBERS OF GENERAL PRACTITIONERS
AND THE CLIENTELE OF PRIMARY HEALTH CARE TEAM
WORKERS

In Chapter One we described the kind of work
associated with the types of community nurse with
which we are concerned. In practice the scope for
development in their roles and organization in the
National Health Service is constrained by the
strength of the available workforce of community
nurses and their workload and trends in these var-
iables (Health Visitors' Association, 1981).

Superficially at least the numbers of whole
time equivalents (w.t.es) of district nurses and
health visitors in England have both shown substantial increases in the period from 1975 to 1979
and subsequently. Thus the Chief Nursing Officer

in her report 'Nursing 1977-80' (DHSS, 1981a) reports a 17.8% increase in the number (w.t.e.) of district nurses (i.e. SRN and SEN with and without district training) from 11,685 to 13,738 in the period 1975 to 1979.* From 1980 the basis on which the numbers of district nurses and health visitors were calculated changed and therefore is not comparable with earlier years. However, the numbers (i.e. on the new basis) for district nurses for 1980 and 1983 were respectively 12,923 and 14,441.** The number of whole time equivalent health visitors increased by 17.3% from 1975 to 1979* (7,655 to 8,983) and on a different basis of calculation from 8,852 in 1980 to 9,681 in 1983**. (These figures were for England only but those quoted in the report of the Royal Commission on the National Health Service (1979) for Great Britain over the period 1967-77 reveal a very similar picture.) The increase in district nursing numbers in the period 1975-79 is almost entirely accounted for by increases in the number (w.t.e.) of SRNs and in particular SRNs with district nurse training. Moreover the increase in the number of ancillary staff (w.t.e.) employed in support of district nursing services during this period was 50%, from just over 2,000 to just over 3,000. (The source of all numbers quoted in this paragraph is the DHSS Primary Health Care Service Statistical Tables 1975-79 and 1980-83.) The increase in the number (w.t.e.) of health visitors between 1975-79* was of course by definition an increase in staff qualified in health visiting. However, the number of supporting staff to health visitors in the community health services (as distinct from the school health services) was relatively small and static.

The number of practice nurses was estimated as 650 (w.t.e.) in 1975 (DHSS, 1975, see page 46 of this book) and 1,100 in 1982 (DHSS, 1982). The steering group of the RCN et al. (1984) reported that there were thought to be about 5,000 practice nurses employed in England (not necessarily all whole time).

---

*Numbers from 1975 onwards include senior grades at area/district.
**Note that the working week for community nurses was reduced from 40 hours to 37½ hours as from April 1981 and the numbers in post after that date should be deflated correspondingly when comparing them with numbers in 1980 and before.

Developments in community nursing since 1974

As to nurses entering training for community nursing, the Chief Nursing Officer (DHSS, 1981a) expressed disappointment at the continuing decline in the number of candidates entering health visitor training. Entrants to district nurse training (SRN and SEN combined) were fewer in the years 1977-80 than in the preceding three years (Standing Medical Advisory Committee and the Standing Nursing and Midwifery Advisory Committee, 1981). (However, in this period major changes in the pattern of district nurse training were under discussion and such training was not at that time mandatory.)

The figures have to be seen in the context of numbers of doctors in general practice. The number increased from 20,377 in 1975 to 21,357 in 1979, and by 1983 to 23,254 with corresponding average list sizes of 2,365 in 1975, 2,286 in 1979 and 2,116 in 1983 (DHSS, 1980a; DHSS, 1985b; DHSS, 1985c).

Thus in short the situation was that in 1983 there was one general practitioner (w.t.e.) per 2,116 of the population, one district nurse* per 3,243** of the population, and one health visitor* per 4,838** of the population. This compares with DHSS targets of one district nurse per 4,000 (2,500 in areas with extensive attachment schemes or a high proportion of elderly and/or disabled people) and one health visitor per 4,300 (3,000 in areas with extensive attachment schemes or high immigrant population) (DHSS, 1972). The Jameson Committee (Ministry of Health, 1956) had proposed one health visitor to about 4,300 population. The British Medical Association has been arguing for one general practitioner per 1,700 of the population (BMA, 1983). However, as the BMA publication pointed out there is a diversity of opinion as to the number of patients that a general practitioner can look after in the community, with appropriate assistance from the nursing and allied professions. (The complexity of this question has been documented in Butler, 1980.) Marsh (in Marsh and Kaim-Caudle, 1976) has argued that if the range of work undertaken by community nurses is increased in line with his suggestions then it would be possible for relatively fewer general practitioners to provide an adequate if not enhanced standard of care if supported by rel-

---

*Using the definitions on which numbers quoted in page 16 are based.
**This is based on population figures taken from DHSS (1984a)

atively more district nurses and health visitors per head of the population. There will clearly be no unequivocal answer to the kinds and quantities of various primary health care providers needed at least until the role and range of duties appropriate to each is defined. However it would appear that the supply of health visitors and district nurses has consistently fallen below 'national norms', arguably to a greater extent than in the case of general practitioners - with shortages particularly acute in some inner city areas (the Acheson Report, London Health Planning Consortium, 1981). Despite the relative shortage of district nurses and health visitors there have, as this book shows, been developments and innovations in community nursing.

ATTACHMENT OF COMMUNITY NURSING STAFF TO GENERAL PRACTITIONERS

Hicks (1976) reported that by 1973 about 75% of community nurses in the National Health Services were attached to general practitioners and that the number of district nurses and health visitors so organized was increasing steadily. Although there was an apparent absence of scientific evaluation of attachment schemes, and some reservations about the costs and benefits especially for health visitors, the assumption was that attachment was here to stay and was desirable.

However by 1981, the report of the Joint Working Group of the Standing Medical Advisory Committee and the Standing Nursing and Midwifery Advisory Committee on the primary health care team (the Harding Report, see Chapter Three) stated 'nurse attachments to general practices are increasingly being reviewed and in the last two years or so a number of health authorities particularly in urban areas have reverted to a geographical pattern of working'. The report suggested various reasons for an apparent growing disenchantment with attachment. These included: shortage of nursing staff; the need to provide a nursing service to the whole community requiring a degree of geographical nurse cover, particularly in areas with a high mobility of population; and the fact that the success of earlier attachment schemes had much to do with their being implemented in areas particularly well suited to attachment by virtue of the existence of group practices serving geographical areas and enthusiastic about primary health care team work, which obscured the fact that attachment could in other circumstances be less effective. Both this report and others which commended attachment, at least as an ideal, emphasized the importance as far as possible of zoning general practice attachment areas so that matching geographical areas for general practitioners and attached community nurses would exist. This would avoid the situation sometimes found in inner cities, whereby numerous practices and attached nurses served patients in the same tower block (see e.g. London Health Planning Consortium, 1981 - the Acheson Report). 'Health Visiting in the 80s' (Health Visitors' Association, 1981) took the view that attachment posed particular problems for health visitors (see page 74 of this book).

Hicks (1976) offered a straightforward definition of attachment, namely 'schemes in which a health visitor or home nurse is responsible for providing services to all patients on lists of all specified general practitioners with whom she has regular consultations. She is not limited to working in a geographical district'. However by 1981 it was argued that attachment needed more precise definition and/or could take various forms with the result that it was sometimes no longer agreed by all the professional parties involved as to whether or not community nursing staff were in fact attached to some practices (See e.g. Hughes and Roberts, 1981).

The appendix to circular CNO(77)8, 'Nursing in Primary Health Care' (DHSS, 1977a), sets out the conditions in which attachment schemes will lead to team work and also the adverse conditions where team work will not have the highest priority (see page 51). The General Medical Services Committee has supported attachment of health visitors and district nurses, and has reservations about the zoning of practice catchment areas (British Medical Journal, 1981, Vol. 283, Supplement, p.1557 and British Medical Journal, 1980, Vol. 281, Supplement, p.166). The Harding Report (Standing Medical Advisory Committee and the Standing Nursing and Midwifery Advisory Committee, 1981) argued that mere attachment for community nursing staff did not imply effective team work though it would probably help, while it was possible that in some circumstances effective team work could take place in the absence of attachment.

For all this, attachment remains the norm for community nurses. 'The Health Service in England,

Annual Report 1984' (DHSS, 1985c) reported that 'over 80% of health visitors and district nurses are now working in close cooperation with family doctors...'. In most circumstances the issue is not so much whether attachments of some kind should continue but how to arrange matters relating to primary health care so that the potential benefits of this approach are fully realized.

FROM HOME NURSE TO DISTRICT NURSE

The National Health Service and Public Health Act of 1968 enabled district nurses and health visitors to work in clinics and not just in patients' homes. This opened the way to the development which Hicks (1976) noted, that by 1973 about half of the contacts recorded by the district nurse with patients took place in treatment rooms of health centres and other primary health care premises. In order for this development to take place, of course it was necessary that there should be suitable clinical accommodation in which district nurses could work, and one consequence of the implementation of the Charter for the Family Doctor Service (British Medical Journal, Supplement, 8th March 1965) was to encourage doctors to work in health centres and other similar premises where such accommodation could be provided. Indeed it seemed at this time that the district nurse would be a natural, if not the only (see below) provider of care in the treatment room of the health centre or general practitioner's premises. By the mid 1980s, with the establishment from late 1981 of a mandatory post basic training course for those becoming district nurses (in the full sense), the importance and distinctive character of this branch of community nursing had been confirmed. However, in a consultative paper on proposed changes in nurse education produced by the English National Board, 1985, it was asserted that 'district nurses report that a growing number of RGNs and SENs are being employed in the community without preparation to meet the increasingly complex need'.

HEALTH VISITING

A number of factors in the last ten years caused health visitors some disquiet and gave rise to a good deal of questioning within the profession as to what the role of health visitors should be and how they should fit into the National Health

Developments in community nursing since 1974

Service organization. These are:

1. The rise of the social work profession, which
    culminated in the transfer under the Local
    Authority Social Services Act 1970 to local
    authority social services departments of some
    work which had hitherto been undertaken by
    health visitors. This meant that certain asp-
    ects of the welfare of young children and
    their families became the responsibility of
    social services departments from which health
    visitors were organizationally separated. Also
    home helps were transferred to social services
    departments.

2. Attachment of health visitors to general prac-
    tices raised questions for both as to the
    nature of the professional relation implied
    and the role of health visiting in relation to
    general practice. Health visitors had tradi-
    tionally had a good deal of autonomy, at least
    as regards general practitioners. The
    emphasis on the counselling and preventive
    work of health visiting was also somewhat
    different from the curative emphasis of gen-
    eral practice (and indeed arguably of other
    attached community nurses).

3. That there was a role for health visitors in
    the care of the increasing number of elderly
    and very elderly, seemed clear, but this was a
    very different group from the principal client
    group of health visitors (young children and
    their mothers) and not one that appealed univ-
    ersally to the profession (Health Visitors'
    Association, 1981). The division of respons-
    ibility between district nurses whose clients
    traditionally included a high proportion of
    these elderly and health visitors was not
    entirely clear.

4. It became progressively evident during the
    seventies that the birth rate had steadily
    declined thus correspondingly reducing the
    number of the health visitors' principal
    clientele.

5. The reorganization of the National Health Ser-
    vice in 1974 set the health visiting service
    firmly within the hierarchical management sys-
    tem of National Health Service nursing gener-

ally. This meant that even within a community
nursing division, the health visitor's superior might not be qualified as a health visit-
or, and certainly the chief nursing officers
(district nursing officers) might well be from
another branch of nursing, given the predominance in terms of sheer numbers of hospital
nurses as compared to community nurses of all
kinds. Subsequent reorganization has not
altered this fundamentally although (see page
8) the hierarchical structure of nursing above
the level of the unit has been weakened, if
not eliminated. Also the arrival of general
managers at unit and district level has introduced a new factor into the management of services, the effects of which for good or ill
remain to be seen.

So for these and maybe other reasons, coupled
with the continuing shortage of health visitors and
potential health visitors (entering training), by
the mid 1980s there was a clear call from the
Health Visitors' Association and the Royal College
of Nursing for a fully research based enquiry into
the role and state of health visiting, to update
and place on a more scientific basis the recommendations and observations of the Jameson Committee
(Ministry of Health, 1956) of thirty years ago.

PRACTICE NURSES

The implementation of the Charter for the
Family Doctor Service (British Medical Journal,
Supplement, 8th March 1965) facilitated the employment by general practitioners of practice nurses,
in that it allowed for 70% reimbursement of cost of
salaries of up to two full-time staff to each practitioner, and such staff might include those with
nursing qualifications. With the spread of attachment schemes for community nurses it seemed possible that district nurses might largely replace
practice nurses on the grounds that the general
practitioner incurred no cost in the case of district nurses attached to his practice. However,
there is evidence that practice nurses were, if
anything, becoming more numerous as time went on
(see page 16). Various reports expressed concern
about relationships between practice nurses and
health authority employed community nurses (see
e.g. the Harding Report, 1981, cited on page 18)
and tended to suggest that it would be desirable in

the long run for practice nurses to be phased out. In contrast the General Medical Services Committee was committed to the position that the direct employment of nurses by general practitioners should be encouraged (British Medical Journal, 1981, Vol. 283, 5th December, Supplement p.1557). The initiative in 1980 of the Royal College of Nursing which led to the formation of a steering group comprising representation of relevant nursing and medical organizations and its subsequent report (see page 93 of this book) arguably suggest a general acceptance of, if not universal enthusiasm for, their continued existence and role.

CHANGING PATTERNS OF ACCOMMODATION FOR PRIMARY HEALTH CARE SERVICES

A number of factors have encouraged family doctors to work in groups from purpose built premises for many years - the group practice allowance*, general economies of scale relating to the employment of ancillary staff and the functioning of buildings, the building of health centres and so on. The idea of purpose built premises for primary health care has been in existence from the outset of the National Health Service and indeed before (see for instance the Dawson Report, Ministry of Health (1920) and the National Health Service Act, 1946), but from the 1960s onwards, considerable changes in general practice took place so that by 1983 76% of doctors (unrestricted principals) were in receipt of group practice allowances (DHSS, 1985b) and the number of health centres had grown to 1,070 involving a quarter of the general practitioners in England. (Numbers of health centres based on the 'Directory of Health Centres', 1984, MMI Publications.)

Since health centres were provided initially by local health authorities, and from 1974 by health authorities, they were natural bases for health authority employed community nursing staff too. Thus there was in health centres generally some form of office accommodation for community

---

* To be in receipt of a group practice allowance it was essential to be practising from suitable shared surgery accommodation in a group of at least three doctors (in rural areas, two were sometimes sufficient). Usually such a group would be in partnership but this was not invariably the case particularly in health centres.

nursing staff, treatment room facilities staffed by
a nurse whether health authority or general practice employed and a common room open to all those
working at or from the health centre, which provided a natural forum for meetings between the general practitioners and those working with them to
provide primary health care, especially district
nurses and health visitors. The common room was
not always much used by all staff particularly if
it was remote from some parts of the health centre.
Clearly, working from the same premises facilitated
communication between community nurses and general
practitioners in comparison with the situation
which the health centre often replaced, of nurses
being based at geographically distinct community
nursing premises and the general practitioners
working from limited domestic scale accommodation.

Purpose built or purpose adapted group practice premises would not, in the nature of things,
normally be designed to include the same range of
accommodation for staff other than the general
practitioners and those directly employed by them,
in contrast to health centres. However, the very
fact that they normally included several consulting
rooms and not infrequently had some form of treatment room and common room facilities, meant that
there was space for meetings between community
nurses and general practitioners. Indeed formally
or informally, community nurses attached to practices might be based at the group practice premises
- though in this case the problem of providing
secretarial and clerical support to the community
nurses could arise even though there was a will to
do so on the part of the health authority.

PRIMARY HEALTH CARE TEAM DEVELOPMENT

Many of the developments described in the last
few sections have in one way or another been concerned with bringing community nurses into closer
working contact with general practitioners but this
does not necessarily bring about teamwork. The
concept of the primary health care team is associated with the way in which they work in relation
to one another, as Hicks (1976) remarks:

> There is no guarantee that if we bring to-
> gether groups of doctors, health visitors,
> nurses, social workers, receptionists and a
> secretariat, they will automatically weld
> themselves into a cohesive combination dir-

ected purposefully to furthering the objectives and goals of primary care. Cooperation
is assured only by persistent and close study.
To hope to get results without intelligent
control of means is to resort to some principle of magic which we all know is ineffec-
tive.

Primary health care is diffuse in its purposes
and objectives - there is so much that is being
done or might be done to prevent illness and allev-
iate symptoms in the community. From the beginning
the National Health Service aimed to bring together
preventive and curative health activities at the
primary level of care, for example in health centres (see section 21 of the National Health Service
Act, 1946 and Ministry of Health, 1946). Unfortunately the original structure of the National Health
Service militated against this in that the general
practitioner service, with its emphasis on cure and
comfort but with a responsibility for named persons
in the community, was organizationally separate
from the preventive services provided by the local
health authority via the Medical Officer of Health
and amongst others health visitors, and from the
home (district) nursing services. This division
between the family practitioner services and the
community nursing services persists in the restruc-
tured National Health Service. Each of these
health service workers, moreover, has their own
specific duties and goals laid down for them and
the overall objectives of primary health care were
not the responsibility, in terms of accountability
for services provided, of any of the potential
members of a primary health care team (see e.g.
Health Visitors' Advisory Group of the Royal
College of Nursing Society of Primary Health Care
Nursing 1984, page 96 of this book). The welding
together into a team of these various providers of
primary care was arguably therefore all the more
important for being problematical.
  The idea of a team approach to primary health
care is far from new and was one of the reasons
behind the movement towards group practice and
health centres described in the last section. However, it seems that team care began to emerge as a
powerful force during the 1960s. The Charter of
the Family Doctor Service (1965) (see page 22) and
the measures to facilitate the spread of group
practice and the building of health centres by both
Conservative and Labour governments, the widespread

adoption of attachment schemes for health visitors
and district nurses, the Public Health Act of 1968
(see page 20), all in various ways made the primary
health care team a realistic option in the National
Health Service. There was much professional support for the idea; thus for example 'Present State
and Future Needs' (College of General Practitioners
1965) contained a chapter on the health team and a
major conference supported by the Royal College of
General Practitioners, the Royal College of Midwives, the Royal College of Nursing, the Queen's
Institute of District Nursing, the Society of Medical Officers of Health, the Health Visitors' Association and the National Association of State
Enrolled Nurses took place in 1967 with the subject
of 'Family health care - the team'. In the 1970s
as 'primary health care' came to be the definitive
term for the actions and purposes of the various
parties involved, there was evidence everywhere of
a growing interest in the team. There was for
example a series of television programmes aimed at
existing and potential teams supported by a book of
essays (Bloomfield and Follis, 1974). The report
of a British Medical Association panel on primary
health care teams (BMA, 1974) listed a number of
advantages of such teamwork for both givers and
receivers of care, namely -

> Care given by a group of those most approp-
> riately qualified is greater than any one in-
> dividual can give and the team approach en-
> ables the proper use to be made of the skills
> of its members and of the resources available
> to them in the community. Peer influence and
> informal learning within the team raise the
> standards of care and improve the corporate
> status of the team within the community, and
> furthermore will make it more likely that the
> team members will find their jobs satisfying.
> Moreover, the team approach encourages health
> education of the patients on a co-ordinated
> basis. The community benefits from a reduct-
> ion in the prevalence of disease and the in-
> dividual from efficient and understanding
> treatment when he is ill.

In the same year a major study by Gilmore,
Bruce and Hunt was published. Entitled 'The Work
of the Nursing Team in General Practice', but much
concerned with the general practitioner as well as
with nurses, it looked into factors affecting the

development of teamwork. In another publication, based on the same fieldwork, 'An Analysis of Factors Influencing Teamwork in General Medical Practice' (Hunt, 1974), a number of theoretical considerations relating to the working of teams in general were considered in relation to the particular context of primary health care.

Successive government publications in the seventies (see next chapter) emphasized the importance of primary health care within the National Health Service and implicitly or explicitly endorsed the idea of the primary health care team, though it was recognized that there were circumstances which made effective teamwork in primary care so difficult as to make the development of such teamwork not of the highest priority. A note of caution too as the effects of working within primary health care teams was sounded by the Health Visitors' Association in both 'Health Visiting in the Seventies' and'Health Visiting in the Eighties' (see page 74 of this book). The terms of reference of the Harding Committee (1981) (see page 80 of this book), are another sign of concern about the primary health care team. The report of the Committee, whilst in no doubt about the importance and value of primary health care teamwork, painted an at times sombre picture of its working out in practice.

The Royal Commission on the National Health Service (1979) commented : 'A recent development of great significance has been the growth of teamwork in primary care ... teamwork in primary care is at an early stage. It will have a major contribution to make to raising standards of service to patients in the community.'

The fact that post basic training is now mandatory for those proposing to follow careers as general practitioners, health visitors and district nurses, offers the possibility of joint education for part of the training, which in some locations is being realized (see e.g. Jones, 1986).

A number of the developments which we shall be describing later in this book (Chapter Four) also mean that in recent years the nursing members of the primary health care team have been able to offer a much more extensive range of caring services to clients and patients of the team; services of a kind which, if they are to be utilized effectively really do require the understanding and cooperation implicit in the idea of a 'team'.

MANAGEMENT ARRANGEMENTS FOR NURSES IN THE NATIONAL HEALTH SERVICE

The report of the Committee on Senior Nursing Staff Structure (the Salmon Report, Ministry of Health, Scottish Home and Health Department, 1966) led to the establishment of an elaborate nursing management structure in hospitals and this had been followed by the report of the Working Party on Management Structure in the Local Authority Nursing Services (the Mayston Report, Department of Health and Social Security, Scottish Home and Health Department, 1969), recommending a similar though simpler structure for community nurses. However the 1974 reorganization of the National Health Service, as a result of which a unified management structure for all health authority employed nurses came into being, brought out the full implications of such a hierarchy for community nursing. This had significance for their professional autonomy and professional relationships within the primary health care team. For better or worse, the nursing officer was an interested party in, but not usually a member of, the primary health care team. She had management responsibilities which included supervising the attachment of her subordinates to general practitioners in relation to the overall goals of the nursing services within the locality for which she was responsible. This sometimes led to difficulties as the Harding Report (Standing Medical Advisory Committee and the Standing Nursing and Midwifery Advisory Committee, 1981) observed:

For example it was said that
i) senior nurses were, on occasion, redeploying nursing staff and in some cases had terminated attachments without consulting beforehand the general practitioners and nurses involved;
ii) nursing staff were being redeployed on a temporary basis to provide cover for colleagues away sick, on holiday or on training courses, at very short notice so that other members of the team had insufficient time to rearrange their working schedules to take account of their colleague's absence and
iii) there were sometimes difficulties arising out of conflict between health authority policy and the general practitioner's expectation of what a nurse should do; for example in the fields of vaccination and immunisation, and of family planning.

Elsewhere the same report recommended that:

constraints that place limits on the range of
duties which health authority employed nurses
may undertake should be subject to periodic
review by health authorities in consultation
with local medical committees along with any
other factors which might prevent attached
nursing staff working alongside general practitioners in surgery-based treatment rooms.

Thus it appears that for good or ill the existence
of a managerial hierarchy within the community
nursing service did enable health authorities to
exercise a greater degree of control over attached
community nursing staff than perhaps was the case
prior to the reorganization of the National Health
Service in 1974. Though the quotations given tend
to see this increased control in a negative light,
it did also enable the community nursing service to
negotiate with general practitioners on more equal
terms than was perhaps previously the case when
district nurses and health visitors were operating
as more autonomous but isolated individuals.
    The 1982 restructuring of the National Health
Service (see the circular HC(80)8, 'Health Service
Development: Structure and Management', DHSS,1980b)
endorsed and continued with the principles under-
lying the organization of nursing established at
the 1974 reorganization. As far as primary health
care services were concerned, however, there was
some anxiety in the professions at the possibility
that there would not be distinct community units,
but rather that these services would be linked in
with other services in units based on, for example,
geographical territories. Thus for instance, the
British Medical Association conference, July 1982,
supported a motion that community services 'should
be encompassed by a single community care unit on
which the general practitioner should be represented as of right' (Health and Social Service
Journal, 1982, Vol. 92, July 15, p.842) and the
Royal College of Nursing, in May 1982, drew the
attention of family practitioner committees 'to the
commitment of the major nursing organizations to a
structure that has a separate unit for community
nursing services in the reorganized National Health
Service' (see e.g. British Medical Journal, 1982,
Vol. 284, Supplement 22 May, p.1584).
    In the event some districts did distribute
community nurses over more than one unit of manage-

ment, though how this arrangement compared with
community units in terms of satisfaction of staff
and effectiveness and efficiency in achieving community service goals is not known. Since then the
Griffiths Report (NHS Management Inquiry, 1983)
which advocated that the NHS itself, regions, districts and units should each be managed by a general manager, has been implemented. At the time of
writing, such officers have been or are being
appointed and where in office are drawing up plans
for management structures within their spheres of
responsibility. The effects of this substitution of
a single manager in place of a team of officers
taking decisions on the basis of consensus have yet
to be seen. General managers came from a variety
of backgrounds, those at district and regional
level mostly appear to have been recruited from the
National Health Service (about 80%) rather than
industry or business and a few (5) were nurses
(Health and Social Services Journal, 1985, Vol. 95,
No. 4964, September 12, Appointments Supplement;
see also leading article p.1113).
    Some aspects of the management of community
nurses remained to be decided. The editorial of
the Family Practitioner Services (Vol. 11, No. 5,
May 1984) observed that 'the possibility of family
practitioner committees rather than health authorities employing district nursing staff and health
visitors has also been raised'. This now, however,
seems unlikely following the publication of the
report by the Community Nursing Review Team (DHSS,
1986) and the discussion paper on family practitioner services (DHSS et al. 1986) (see pages 101-9
respectively). Interestingly the Health and Social
Security Act (1984) stipulated that one member of
the family practitioner committee must be 'a district nurse, midwife or health visitor (appropriately registered) and who has recent experience
of providing services to patients (other than patients resident in hospital) in any such capacity'.

HEALTH SERVICE PRIORITIES AND THE LIMITS AND COSTS
OF MEDICINE

    Scientific medicine as a dominating and all
conquering force in the restoration and preserva-
tion of health, has come under attack from writers
such as Illich (see e.g. Illich, 1976). Nursing
was largely exempt by its nature from such criticisms. Moreover during the seventies priorities
within the National Health Service were increas-

ingly centred on groups such as the frail elderly,
the mentally ill and the mentally and physically
handicapped (DHSS, 1976 and 1977b) - areas where
medicine could offer relatively little by way of
cure and where carefully planned and organized and
compassionate nursing care was at least as important. Particularly in the case of the elderly, the
priority arose largely because there was a steadily
increasing need for care for such people, as more
and more of the population were aged 75 years or
more.

There has also been a trend in policy towards
'community care' interpreted broadly as the shift-
ing of care of patients where possible from hospitals to institutions in the community or to patients' homes (e.g. DHSS, 1976 and 1981b). Such a
trend clearly has implications for caring professions in the community such as community nurses.
This was explicitly recognized (DHSS 1976) in recommending a fairly rapid increase in the numbers of
district nurses and health visitors - a growth rate
of 6% per annum was proposed.

The efficacy of scientific medicine came under
attack at a time when its costs were escalating to
an extent which caused concern to even the wealth-
iest nations. Hence there has been a revived
interest in health education and self care, the
former being an area in which health visitors have
been particularly concerned.

Questions of cost and availability of trained
doctors have led to the emergence, in developed and
developing countries throughout the world, of new
types of health personnel, intermediate in role
between doctors and nurses. Hence for example the
emergence of the 'bare foot' doctor in China on the
one hand and the nurse practitioner and the physician's assistant in the United States of America.
This development in the USA had been noted in the
literature from the late 1960s onwards and Hicks
(1976) drew attention to a model evaluative study
comparing doctors in a group practice in Burlington, Canada, with nurse practitioners, as the persons of first contact for patients of the practice
(Spitzer et al. 1974). There has been some interest in such developments in the United Kingdom. The
British Medical Association (BMA, 1974), whilst
favouring some development in the role of the nurse
in primary health care, felt there was no necessity
at that time for a worker of the physician's-
assistant type in the National Health Service.

Reedy (1978) subsequently described developments in the USA. As yet there have been few
experiments in the United Kingdom concerning the
impact of nurse-practitioner type staff. (We refer
to those we have identified in Chapter Four.)

One of the central issues in the development
of an extended role of this kind is whether, if at
all, such practitioners could prescribe drugs. That
it was reasonable for a nurse to do so, within appropriately defined limits, was suggested by the
existing practice of midwives. (See also the Royal
College of Nursing report of a working party of the
Royal College of Nursing Family Planning Nurses
Forum, 'Nurse Prescribers of Oral Contraceptives
for the Well-woman', RCN, 1980, where it was proposed that family planning nurses should so
prescribe.)

MEMBERSHIP OF THE EUROPEAN ECONOMIC COMMUNITY AND
WORLD HEALTH ORGANIZATION

The period covered by this review coincides
with most of the period during which the United
Kingdom has been a member of the EEC. The United
Kingdom became a member on 1st January 1973. There
has been some direct impact from EEC membership,
for example as member nations move towards mutual
acceptability of one another's medical and nursing
qualifications. One consequence of this has been
the definition of a practising nurse which could
exclude some practising health visitors (EEC,
Nursing Directive 77/452/EEC). Also directive
77/453/EEC was concerned with training and among
other things required that the training of nurses
should include experience of primary health care
nursing or at least home nursing.

Membership of the EEC has arguably had a more
general effect of causing organizations in health
services as in other spheres of life to adopt a
European perspective. The World Health Organization offers another forum for discussion of health
services and health care problems at an international level, and following the Alma Ata Declara-
tion (WHO, 1978) the crucial role of primary
health care in improving the level of health of the
population of member nations has been emphasized.
It would be wrong to suggest that either the EEC or
WHO exert a profound effect on the day-to-day
running of community nursing activities in the
United Kingdom but they do offer the innovator in
this field a wide range of experience upon which to

draw for ideas, and for the justification of developments. (See for example Hockey, 1983 and also
page 78 of this book.)

INFORMATION FOR AND ABOUT NURSING: THE NURSING
PROCESS, KÖRNER, RECORD SYSTEMS FOR COMMUNITY
NURSING AND COMPUTERS

Health visitors and district nurses have long
been required to return certain basic information
about clients seen for local and national statistical purposes and to keep records about various
clients to enable nursing care to proceed. One
issue is the question of access to general practitioners' records and the possibility of entering
information by community nurses on to these in relation to clients/patients attended. Several developments have had some bearing on these matters in
the last decade or so.

a)   The nursing process
     Central to 'the nursing process' is the idea
that the nurse would be responsible for all aspects
of nursing care for an individual patient (at least
whilst on duty) rather than merely undertaking
specific nursing tasks as prescribed by a doctor or
some superior nurse.

     It is a method by which nurses can move
towards planning more individualised care and
evaluating the care which has been given'
(Royal College of Nursing, 1979).
     The process involves the four stages of
gathering information, planning care, perform-
ing the nursing care as planned, evaluating
the care given. The process is continuous and
cyclical. (Baly, 1980.)

     To enable the nurse to plan care, she would
obtain the necessary information by completing a
questionnaire which covered social and psychological factors relating to the care of the patient as
well as more basic information relevant to the
technical nursing of the patient's particular condition (which would then be updated as the care pro-
ceeded). The health visitor and district nurse
would historically have been much more likely to
look after, in total, the care of the patient/cli-
ent referred to them than would a hospital nurse,
so the application of the nursing process to community nursing would come more naturally; though of

course the kind of information collected and the discipline of carrying out the various stages of the process may have been novel. At all events the nursing process implied maintaining more extensive information about the patient than had previously been the case and a new evaluation of information. A number of articles on the nursing process have appeared since 1975 (see for example the bibliography in RCN, 1979). Examples of recent articles on the nursing process relating to district nursing and health visiting respectively are Ellis (1985) and Clark (1985).

b) The Körner recommendations
The Steering Group on Health Services Information (Chairman Mrs E Korner) was appointed by the Secretary of State for Social Services in February 1980 with the following objectives (Steering Group on Health Services Information, NHS/DHSS, 1982):

1) to agree, implement and keep under review principles and procedures to guide the future development of health services information systems;
2) to identify and resolve health services information issues requiring a co-ordinated approach;
3) to review existing health services information systems; and
4) to consider proposals for changes to, or developments in, health services information systems arising elsewhere and if acceptable, to assess priorities for their development and implementation.

The steering group produced a number of reports each covering a part of the National Health Service. The Fifth Report was devoted to community health services (Steering Group on Health Services Information, NHS/DHSS, 1984). The steering group in this report as in others identified a minimum data set* for various purposes. The Fifth Report discussed information:

---

*'The minimum data set is defined as the data without which a health authority and its management team would be handicapped in the discharge of their duty to plan, monitor and account for the services for which they are responsible.' (Steering Group on Health Services Information, NHS/DHSS 1984.)

i) about services <u>to</u> the community (these are
    'services of prevention or intervention which
    are provided as a matter of public policy
    rather than in response to individual demands
    for treatment or care', Steering Group on
    Health Services Information, NHS/DHSS, 1984);
ii) about patient care <u>in</u> the community (this 'is
    the treatment or ca<u>re</u> outside hospital of pat-
    ients with identified physical or mental ill-
    ness or disability', Steering Group on Health
    Services Information, NHS/DHSS, 1984);
iii) information for operational management (essen-
    tially information about patterns of work and
    workload).

The government resolved (see parliamentary
statement April 1984 by John Patten and accompanying circular HC(84)10, DHSS, 1984b) that the
recommendations of the Körner Group should be
implemented within the National Health Service
mostly by April 1987 and the remainder by April
1988 (British Journal of Health Care Computing,
1984 Vol. 1, No. 2, p.5). This imposed on those
developing information systems a duty to make sure
that the Körner minimum data sets relating to any
aspects of the NHS were included in any arrangements they set up. Some examples of this kind of
activity with a community nursing component are:

i) The Financial Information Project (FIP, South
    Birmingham Health Authority) which includes a
    patient based computerized record system for
    home nursing integrated with a loan of equip-
    ment system. It also includes a domiciliary
    incontinence system and will include a geriat-
    ric health visiting system. (See Catchpole,
    1985a,b and Saddington, 1984.)
ii) The Management Information Pilot Project
    (MIPP) which has been piloted in the Broms-
    grove and Redditch Health Authority. This
    covers all levels and types of staff, from
    district nurses through to mental handicap
    nurses. (See Catchpole, 1985a,b.) The hard-
    ware used for this community module will
    additionally provide remote data entry fac-
    ilities for the National Standard Child Health
    System running on the regional main frame.

c) Computing and community nursing
    The decade with which we are concerned has
been one of substantial and accelerating develop-

ments in computers and associated facilities. One of the most striking recent developments has been that of cheap, relatively portable, but by the standards of even a few years ago, enormously powerful micro-computing facilities. They are moreover relatively easy to use, attractive for planning and audit and other purposes by non-specialists in computing because of the increasingly wide range of 'user friendly' software available. Additionally, whilst these microcomputers can by themselves prove powerful tools for data storage and processing, they can be linked in various ways with one another and with one or more mainframe computers to inter-communicate. So for example a district micro-computer can 'send' relevant sections of part-processed data to a regional computer and receive useful district-specific information from the mainframe for incorporation in its local data set for local analysis.

Catchpole (1985b) has provided an authoritative report on the application of computers in the community health services based on a survey addressed in the first instance in November 1984 to chief nursing officers of district health authorities. His survey reveals the way in which a variety of information systems relevant to community nursing have been developed over the years. They include (as well as those mentioned in the preceding section): the Leicester Community Health System in operation since 1973, which maintains basic records for each patient of the district nurses in the authority and amongst other things produces a daily visit schedule for each nurse to work to as well as management information; the National Standard Child Health System currently in use in more than half of the authorities in the country - the system consists of several modules; a child register, immunization module, pre-school health module, school health module and statistical module (all but the first are optional); other systems for the maintenance of registers and recall systems; stock control systems; a sophisticated statistical reporting system on the characteristics of patients and workload associated with them (e.g. the Wessex Regional Community Nursing System), to mention but a few.

These systems operate on a variety of computer systems, ranging from small stand-alone micro-computers to systems of micro-computers of varying power, linked up to a central regional mainframe computer.

Even quite small privately owned computers can
be of use. Sturgeon (1983) for example reports the
use of the family's home computer to plan a district nurse's visiting schedule. Parkinson (1983)
speculates on the use by district nurses of hand-
held battery terminals on which information can be
stored in a form (e.g. micro-cassettes) which can
then be processed by a centrally based computer.
The nurses would take one of these terminals with
them on their visiting rounds. The combination of
computing and communication facilities may well
mean that data on patients can be transmitted directly, perhaps from the home in the not too distant
future, by a community nurse in the course of her
visiting, and processed information can be returned
to her so that she can plan the care or advice she
provides accordingly, possibly extending the range
of help that she is in a position to give to patients and clients.

The developments relating to community nurses
have not just been done by others for nurses. There
is evidence of the active interest of the nursing
profession in computing (see for example Scholes et
al. 1983, the report of an international workshop
on the impact of computers on nursing) and the
existence of a British Computer Society Nursing
Specialist Group.

Computing developments in community nursing
relating to primary health care teams cannot be
considered of course in isolation from those in
general practice, and there have been a number of
instances where general practice information has
been put onto a computer. These have included
summaries or sometimes more extensive transcripts
of information on patients' records as well as
purely administrative information relating to the
running of practices, appointment systems etc., and
age/sex and other registers of at risk patients.
The Exeter Primary Health Care Computer Project
(see for example Catchpole, 1985b) attempts to provide an integrated health care system where information collected about a patient's contacts with
his/her general practitioner or other member of the
primary health care team is stored on computer and
made available as required at other points of contact at which care is provided. This project initially used VDU-type terminals linked to a mainframe
computer and more recently has been modified to run
on stand-alone micro-computer systems.

In addition a number of general practitioners
have acquired their own micro-computers for various

purposes, mainly for administration within their practices. The figure was thought to be around 400 practices in 1985 (see Hayes, 1985). The DHSS via the 'micros for GPs scheme' (DHSS, 1985a) has provided 150 general practices involving some 500 or more doctors in the United Kingdom with microcomputer systems to stimulate and evaluate applications of this technology in general practice.

Moreover steps are being taken (see Fisher, 1985) to computerize the records held by family practitioner committees which include those relating to general practitioners in contract with them. Most are based on the implementation of a system developed by the Exeter FPS Computer Unit.

Clearly, given the general practitioner's vital role as the holder of a medical history of the patient from birth onwards, the development of suitable means for storing and processing this information is particularly important although difficulties could arise because each practice is an independent contractor in relation to the NHS, and not part of a bureaucratic system. The importance of such information to district health authorities, if it was available via computer links acceptable to both health authority and general practitioner, and indeed similar links with the FPC, is very considerable. It may well be here in the medium term that the most dramatic development will take place. Community nurses as part of primary health care teams would clearly derive help from any such developments in this direction.

HIGHER AND FURTHER EDUCATION IN NURSING

The management structure for nursing adopted in the 1974 reorganization of the National Health Service was a sign and a means of giving practical effect to the enhanced status of nursing within the service - as an important function closely related to medicine but managerially and to a degree philosophically and technically independent from it. Another sign of and factor promoting the enhancement of nursing status was the emergence of university and polytechnic departments of nursing training nurses who would be graduates, and producing a small but growing number of nurses with higher degrees. The first university department of nursing studies in the United Kingdom had been set up in 1956 in the University of Edinburgh, offering courses leading to a degree in social science and nursing. Gradually other universities followed suit

so that by 1979 there were ten schemes leading to a
university degree in nursing (and others leading to
a CNAA degree) plus registration (Baly, 1980). The
founding of the Journal of Advanced Nursing in
1976, and its continuation to the present with a
style and content which specifically proclaimed its
intention to be numbered with the learned journals
rather than with the professional magazines, is one
indication of the influence and interests of the
academically trained nurses and the academic section of nursing education.

A characteristic of science generally which is
manifested within medicine in particular is increasing specialization, and as nursing has emerged as
a distinct discipline, so

> it is now accepted that some nurses by study-
> ing and research can develop special skills in
> aspects of nursing, for example, terminal care
> stoma care and oncology, and that such nurses
> can be used to advise their colleagues both in
> hospital and community and to play a part in
> teaching other disciplines (Baly, 1980).

Evidence of developments in this direction
included the setting up in 1970 'after much pressure from the Royal College of Nursing', of the
Joint Board of Clinical Nursing Studies (Baly,
1980) which 'has introduced a range of post basic
clinical courses, of a nationally approved standard' (RCN, 1976). Indeed the Royal College of
Nursing in 1971 put forward the concept of the
clinical nurse specialist/consultant in its
evidence to the Committee on Nursing (DHSS, SHHD
and Welsh Office, 1972) (see page 48). A working
party of the Royal College of Nursing set up for
the purpose of identifying the role of the clinical
nurse consultant, establishing her relationship
with other persons in the health service, and
preparation for this role, submitted its findings
to the Committee on Nursing as supplementary
evidence. A subsequent publication 'New Horizons
in Clinical Nursing', (the report of a seminar held
at Leeds Castle in 1975 under the auspices of the
Royal College of Nursing, RCN, 1976) ranged over a
number of aspects of developments of the nursing
role drawing a distinction between the clinical
nurse specialist and the clinical nurse consultant:

> The clinical nurse consultant role was the
> ultimate in clinical nursing requiring know-

ledge in breadth as well as in depth even though clinical expertise might be related to one specialty. A clinical nurse specialist role could be identified, of a more limited nature but, nevertheless of significance in advancing the contribution of the nurse in the care of patients in a particular specialty or with particular needs. Other roles developed by nurses were of an even more specialist nature and might not necessarily require a nursing base on which to build, eg. the nurse therapist role.

The increasing complexity of primary health care has led to the conviction that personnel should be given appropriate training before they become fully accredited operators within this field. Thus in the case of medicine, a period of training has now become mandatory (in effect from February 1981) before a doctor can become a principal in general practice, and likewise it has now become mandatory for district nurses to complete a period of training before they may enter this branch of their profession, as it was already in the case of health visitors (see page 20).

The proposals recently circulated for consultation by the United Kingdom Central Council for Nursing, Midwifery and Health Visiting (UKCC, 1986) regarding the whole range of professional training of nurses from basic registration to the highest specialist and other qualifications will if implemented have a bearing on the status of nursing. This is because it is based on the premise of a single initial professional grade (the registered general nurse) supported by aides, training not being provided in the future for the state enrolled grade. Moreover training for the first registration and indeed higher qualifications (as they are already), will, if these proposals are implemented, be located at higher or further education institutions, particularly in the first year, rather than using the existing apprenticeship type approach. Minimum education qualifications of entry to training for the register are also being raised.

After a common foundation programme of two years, it was proposed that there should be five branches leading to first registration - mental illness, mental handicap, nursing of adults, nursing of children and midwifery. Nurses qualified to the level of first registration would be able to practise in hospital or community settings but

would be led by specialist practitioners with re-
cordable qualifications in the case of community
nursing, in district nursing, community psychiatric
nursing and community mental health nursing; the
health visitor would also be a specialist with re-
cordable qualifications.

Arguably all these developments fit in with
the general philosophy of the nursing process and
will increase the chance of its being creatively
and effectively implemented throughout the NHS.

OTHER MATTERS RELATING TO THE STATUS OF NURSES

Other developments that have some bearing on
the status of nursing (including some already discussed) are:

1. The coming into being of the United Kingdom
   Central Council for Nursing, Midwifery and
   Health Visiting and the associated national
   boards in 1983, as the means of regulating the
   nursing profession including education and
   training, had for those in the community some
   controversial aspects. The UKCC, as the central body is known, is a policy making body
   responsible for the registration, training and
   professional conduct of all nurses, midwives
   and health visitors in the United Kingdom.
   National boards (English, Welsh, Scottish and
   Northern Irish) will be primarily responsible
   for the education and training of nurses, midwives and health visitors within the policies
   made by the UKCC. Decisions made by the UKCC
   and national boards will also affect such matters as continuing education, entitlement to
   practise and registration fees. (These observations are quoted from the document 'How the
   UKCC and four national boards will affect
   you', a large and undated advertisement provided by the UKCC.) The UKCC and the four
   national boards replaced the following bodies

       The General Nursing Council for England
       and Wales
       The General Nursing Council for Scotland
       The Central Midwives Board
       The Central Midwives Board for Scotland
       The Northern Ireland Council for Nurses
       and Midwives
       The Council for the Education and
       Training of Health Visitors

The Joint Board of Clinical Nursing
Studies
The Committee for Clinical Nursing
Studies
The Panel of Assessors for District Nurse
Training

Thus it will be seen that midwifery was
separately regulated and there existed a separate council for the education and training
of health visitors and a panel of assessors
for district nurse training. The 1979 Act
required the UKCC and the national boards, to
each establish a finance committee and a midwifery committee. The latter was to be consulted by the UKCC and national boards on all
matters relating to midwifery functions.
Moreover there was to be a health visiting
joint committee of the UKCC and national
boards, to be consulted by the UKCC and national boards on all matters relating to their
health visiting functions. Initially, such a
committee was not proposed for district nursing. However, in May 1982 in the second consultation paper, working group five which was
concerned with standing and joint committees
proposed the establishment of a district nurse
joint committee and indeed this was implemented. The district nursing joint committee
was to be consulted by the UKCC and the national boards on all matters relating to their
district nursing functions.
It remains to be seen what will be the
impact of these changes on the status and role
of those engaged in community nursing. What
is certain is that both midwifery and health
visiting are now seen as being firmly located
within nursing.

2. The setting up of an individual review body to
recommend salary levels for nursing and professions supplementary to medicine (i.e.organ-
izationally akin to that in operation for the
medical profession within the National Health
Service) might be said to again represent an
enhancement in the status of nursing.

3. As already mentioned, the requirement is that
a community nurse should be a member of each
family practitioner committee (see page 30).
Arguably this represents an enhancement of the

status of community nurses given the present functions of FPCs, and could of course acquire added importance if FPCs were in some way to take on responsibility for community nursing, in which case presumably some increase in representation of that group would be needed.

4. The proposal that the RCGP should admit to affiliate membership non-medical members of the primary health care team, including nurses, is a sign of the recognition of the importance of the contribution such staff make (Nursing Times, Vol. 81, January 2, page 7, 1985).

5. New management arrangements now being implemented (see page 30) represent a challenge, if not a threat, and an opportunity to health care professions, particularly nurses.

Chapter Three

SIGNIFICANT DHSS AND PROFESSIONAL REPORTS AND
POLICY STATEMENTS RELEVANT TO THE DEVELOPMENT OF
COMMUNITY NURSING IN THE LAST DECADE

In this chapter we summarize and quote from
those documents or sections of documents published
since 1974, which are relevant to the community
nursing services as we have defined them. The summaries are in order of their year of publication.
(For similar earlier documents see Hicks, 1976 and
Baly, 1980.) Each document is headed by its title
with the author and year of publication in brackets

1. PRIMARY HEALTH CARE TEAMS - Report of a Panel
(Board of Science and Education of the British Medical Association, 1974).

This report saw the development of primary
health care teams of suitable size (facilitated
also by the movement from single-handed to group
practice by general practitioners) as allowing
improved comprehensive care both by day and by
night. Continuity of care was seen as care for the
patient and the patient's family by one or other
member of the same primary health care team, even
though the choice of doctor would remain an essential right of the patient as between the general
practitioners in the team. It saw the attachment
of the community nurse to general practitioners as
vital so that these staff would serve populations
defined not by geographical district but by patients on the doctor's list. (However, the report
does state that as far as possible overlap between
neighbouring teams should be avoided.) The report
noted that the nursing functions formed three categories at present represented by the health visit-
or the midwife and the district nurse. (It did not
consider practice nurses.) The panel was divided
as to whether curative and preventive functions
could be combined in the same nurse. New training

structures which were evolving were expected to
reallocate functions between registered and enrolled nurses so that each would carry out the functions most appropriate to her abilities. Each
should be trained more specifically for a community
role. The panel considered that the general practitioner was to some degree concerned in all aspects
of primary health care and would therefore act in
an advisory and consultative capacity when necessary within the team. In the clinical sphere he/
she takes the ultimate responsibility, but all
members of the team are free to initiate, and are
responsible for activities within their own fields.
    In certain defined areas, the report concluded
that with appropriate training, registered nurses
could undertake patient assessment and counselling
and in certain circumstances the initiation of therapy. Further study in this area was recommended,
in particular a controlled trial to compare primary
health care teams where the nurse makes independent
decisions in certain areas with those teams where
she does not. It was noted that the midwife already took such independent decisions within her
own sphere of competence. The report discussed
'the possible introduction of a non-professional
grade - an assistant to the physician into the membership of the team', under the general heading of
'Medical Assistant (Feldscher, Medex, Nurse Practitioner, etc.)'. The panel concluded that in the
United Kingdom there was no immediate necessity for
such a grade. The overlap between the duties and
functions of the health visitor and those of the
social worker was noted to be considerable and it
was suggested that the training of both professions
should reflect the complementary nature of their
respective skills and functions so that harmonious
relationships were built up within the team for the
benefit of the patient.

2. NURSING IN GENERAL PRACTICE IN THE REORGANIZED
NATIONAL HEALTH SERVICE - Report of a Joint Working
Party (Royal College of Nursing and the Royal Coll-
ege of General Practitioners, 1974).

    This report confined itself to considering
district nurses and enrolled nurses employed by the
area health authorities who worked mainly in the
homes of patients, and nurses employed by general
practitioners. It noted that despite the widespread development of schemes of attachment of
health authority employed nurses in general pract-

ice, practice employed nurses also appeared to be
increasing, and it pressed for the integration of
general practitioner employed nurses into the nursing team so that they shared cover as far as possible and were not seen as competing agencies; and
also so that they had the same access to educational opportunities as health authority nurses.
The report specifically recommended the establishment of evening and night nursing services in
the community as a means of ensuring continuity in
the provision of nursing services. It gave guarded
approval to the extending of the nurses' role by
taking on some of the tasks seen hitherto to be in
the province of the general practitioner. It emphasized the importance of such tasks being allocated
only to suitably competent and mature nurses and
the need for further training both for such work in
the treatment room and for work in the patient's
home which the committee thought had distinctive
characteristics. The committee distinguished between the straightforward 'triage' function (sorting
the patients into those whom the nurse can treat
and those who should be referred to the doctor) and
the process of 'differential diagnosis'. The need
for the evaluation of any extension of the nurses'
role was emphasized. The report urged that all
nurses working in general practice should be able
to recognize serious psychiatric morbidity and
emotional disturbances and know how to deal most
appropriately with this kind of problem. In several places the report drew attention to the importance of having a nursing perspective on the planning of premises and services and in the formation
of practice policy.

3. NURSES EMPLOYED PRIVATELY BY GENERAL MEDICAL
PRACTITIONERS (Practice Nurses), Staff Training
Memorandum STM(75)13 (DHSS, 1975).

This memorandum contained the following information and advice on practice nurses:

1. As health authorities may be aware, a number
of general medical practitioners providing
general medical services employ qualified
nurses to assist them in their work. They are
usually referred to as "practice nurses" and
are employed mainly within the practice premises or health centres although they may visit
their employers' patients in their homes as
requested. They often work alongside district

nurses and health visitors who form part of the primary health care team. The number of practice nurses in England at present is about 650 (WTE) compared with a total field force of 10,200 (WTE) home nurses. In addition there are some practice nurses who combine nursing with other duties, e.g. receptionist.

2. The effect which the development of primary health care teams will have on the role of the practice nurse and the numbers likely to be employed is not yet clear and consideration of long-term training arrangements required must depend on how the role develops. In the meantime it is desirable that facilities should be available for the refresher training and updating of professional knowledge of the practice nurses employed at present. As part of these arrangements area health authorities who provide in-service education and training for their own community based nurses are asked to consider inviting practice nurses in their area to participate, without charge, including visits of observation etc. to hospitals and other institutions. Suitable forms of education and training would include short courses on specialised topics or techniques, lectures, seminars, discussion groups and periodical staff conferences. Attendance of particular nurses would, of course, be subject to approval by their employers.

3. Travelling and other expenses would be the responsibility of the practice nurse and her employer and it is expected that she would continue to receive her normal salary during the short periods of absence. Area health authorities are asked to bring this Memorandum to the attention of their Family Practitioner Committees and notify them of what facilities are available so that they may in turn inform general medical practitioners in their area who employ practice nurses.

4. PRIORITIES FOR HEALTH AND PERSONAL SOCIAL SERVICES IN ENGLAND. A CONSULTATIVE DOCUMENT (DHSS, 1976a).

This consultative document proposed that district nurse and health visitor numbers should increase at the rate of 6% per annum. In the case of

district nurses this was to provide care for the
increasing number of elderly people in the community; to enable children to be treated as far as
possible in their own homes rather than in hospital; and to look after the younger physically
handicapped outside hospitals. In the case of
health visitors the increase was to allow for improvements in child health and welfare and to give
support to mothers and particularly to protect the
health of the most vulnerable children in the community. (Health visitors were stated to have a crucial role in the prevention of non-accidental injury to children.) It was also to assist in the
care of the increasing number of elderly in the
community.

5.   NEW HORIZONS IN CLINICAL NURSING (Royal College of Nursing of the United Kingdom, 1976).

We have already mentioned this report of a
seminar in Chapter Two as being particularly
concerned with the development of the clinical
nurse specialist/consultant. In Appendix A of the
report, relevant extracts of the Royal College of
Nursing evidence to the Committee on Nursing (DHSS,
Scottish Home and Health Department, Welsh Office,
1972) are listed. This is concerned with post
basic nursing education and career progression.
Here there is a section on nursing in the community
as follows:

> The nurse who opted to work in the com-
> munity setting would be required to obtain the
> post basic credit or credits relevant to com-
> munity nursing, the course of training requir-
> ed for the health visitor and that required
> for the district nurse would both come under
> this head. The nurse would then be equipped
> to practise in the community as a member of
> the community health team. All those services
> at present provided within the community by
> persons required to hold a nursing qualifica-
> tion are included in the term 'community nur-
> sing', and all persons so qualified would be
> members of the 'community health team'. It is
> considered that the desirable organisation of
> community work is that of the Group Practice
> team and further that there is need for an
> increase in the number of health centres on
> which these teams would be based.

Specialisation is not the prerogative of institutional care; it applies also in the community service. Nurses working in the community not infrequently specialise in a particular type of work and are recognised as capable of advising their colleagues in relation to this specialty. This advanced expertize should be supported by further studies, to be defined, and recognised posts should be created at a consultant level; these would parallel the development proposed in the institutional setting.

The 'development proposed' was

that the full contribution of the nurse/midwife as a clinical expert of a high order must be further exploited by identifying a career for her in clinical nursing... This should take the form of creating posts for "clinical nurse consultants" who would work alongside medical consultants. The "Cogwheel" division structure opens up the way for such appointments. Eligibility for these posts would require the possession of qualifications at an advanced level: The Diploma in Nursing would be an appropriate qualification and others might well become available... Needless to say the post of "clinical nurse consultant" should attract salary recognition consistent with the level of responsibility and the high degree of expertise inherent in it.

6. HEALTH SERVICES MANAGEMENT: VACCINATION AND IMMUNISATION - INVOLVEMENT OF NURSING STAFF Circular HC(76)26 (DHSS, 1976b).

The purpose of this circular was to clarify the role of nurses in vaccination and immunization programmes. It stated that:

Authorities should aim to involve nursing staff in vaccination programmes to the extent which best promotes in their local circumstances the objectives of such programmes, viz to achieve maximum acceptance of recommended vaccines at recommended intervals by those members of the population who would benefit while ensuring all necessary safety precautions such as the scrupulous observance of contra-indications.

A doctor engaged in clinical medicine is responsible for all vaccinations, i.e. for the decision as to the suitability of the patient, the appropriate vaccine and its safe administration. While retaining that responsibility, he may delegate all these aspects to a nurse who is willing to be professionally answerable for this work, and who has been approved for the purpose by the employing authority. The delegation may cover an individual patient or a specifically defined group of patients provided that suitable policies and definitions have been drawn up and agreed in advance.

7. FIT FOR THE FUTURE: THE REPORT OF THE COMMITTEE ON CHILD HEALTH SERVICES (DHSS, Department of Education and Science, and Welsh Office, 1976).

The report proposed that within the community nursing service there should be a distinct group of nurses called child health visitors (CHVs) who would have preventive and curative responsibilities in respect of their patients, and who would work in close association with general practitioner paediatricians (general practitioners who would have a special interest in and training in paediatrics). Child health visitors would at least initially be drawn from the ranks of the existing health visitors who would, however, require additional training. The report envisaged that the CHVs would be assisted by child health nurses who would have paediatric training. Thus this report was in a sense adopting a 'McKeownist' approach to nursing care, identifying one group of nurses as being responsible for the preventive and curative nursing care of those under 16 years of age and (by implication, though this was not the function of the report) other groups of nurses similarly concerned with other age groups.

8. PRIORITIES IN THE HEALTH AND SOCIAL SERVICES. THE WAY FORWARD (DHSS, 1977d).

This discussion paper restated the government's intention to increase expenditure on health visiting and district nursing services by 6% per annum. In an appendix on 'more effective uses of NHS resources', among the examples quoted were:

The time that community nursing staff spend on professional duties can be increased when general practitioners practise within defined geographical areas.

...The introduction of a community night nursing service allows patients who are terminally ill or who might otherwise require hospital beds to remain at home. Where such a service is operating, it might be hospital based in order fully to utilise the nursing time and improve communications.

9. NURSING IN PRIMARY HEALTH CARE. Appendix to Circular CNO(77)8 (DHSS, 1977c).

This paper represented an updating of guidance in the light of the report of the Court Committee (DHSS, DES and Welsh Office, 1976) (see page 50 of this chapter) and the consultative document 'Priorties for Health and Personal Social Services in England',(DHSS, 1976a)(see page 47 of this chapter) which in particular gave emphasis to the encouragement of the development of primary health care teams.

It states that experience has shown that where health visiting and district nursing staff have been attached to general practice and have developed cooperative patterns of working, with each discipline providing its own specific skills, the quality of service to individual patients and to families has improved. It has been possible to develop preventive and educative services as well as meeting the clinical needs of the practice population. It is asserted that communications between the various members of the primary health care team and between the primary health care services and other National Health Service and local authority and voluntary services have also been improved.

The attachment of nursing staff to general practice was seen as desirable but not of itself sufficient to create effective primary health care teamwork. The participants in the team have to be sufficiently knowledgeable and motivated if effective teamwork is to take place.

The paper identified certain circumstances where the development of primary health care teams does not assume the highest priority, namely:

a.   where the numbers of nursing staff employed (by the health authority) are insufficient;
b.   where general practitioners do not accept this concept of care;

c   where there is a predominance of single handed general practitioners;

d.   where it is impossible to provide adequate accommodation to enable staff of different professions to work from the same premises;

e.   where there is considerable overlap of the geographical areas covered by general practitioners;

f.   in inner city areas where there are special health and social problems.

Where these conditions apply, however, the development of appropriate patterns of co-operative working remains nevertheless a high priority.

The roles of various kinds of community nurse are then defined and in particular we have already quoted on pages 2-4, those of the nurses relevant to this book, namely the health visitor, the district nurse, treatment room nurse and practice nurse.

The paper states that:

Developments such as early discharge from hospital or day surgery will have implications for primary health care, meaning for example the importance of establishing a 24-hour nursing service in order to provide continuity of care. They will also increase the need for more effective communications between the specialist and primary health care services. ....in practical terms this could be achieved by developing direct channels of communication between health visitors and district nurses and the appropriate ward sisters in hospitals. .....Where nurses with a special knowledge of the care of a particular illness or type of patient (e.g. the physically handicapped, chronically sick children, the mentally ill or the mentally handicapped) work with patients and families in the community and liaise with and advise members of the primary health care team, it is essential that they maintain their expertise, and therefore desirable that they should be based within their specialist field.

10. RESIDENTIAL HOMES FOR THE ELDERLY. ARRANGE-
MENTS FOR HEALTH CARE. A memorandum of guidance.
(DHSS and Welsh Office, 1977).

The following items in this memorandum relate
to the role of primary health care services, in
relation to persons living in residential homes for
the elderly:

Responsibility for the provision of
health care rests in the first instance on the
primary health care services, which can also
contribute to improving the quality of life in
old people's Homes by way of advice and guidance to residents and staff.
...When in the opinion of their general
practitioners residents require professional
nursing care within the Home, this should
wherever possible be provided by nurses employed by the AHA. The nurses will normally be
those working with the doctors who attend the
residents unless some other local arrangement
appears appropriate. In some areas district
nurses are already helping care staff towards
an understanding of the ageing process and
illnesses associated with old age, and where
resources permit, health visitors may also be
involved.
...Caring for dying residents places
extra strain on the staff, and the head of the
Home should be encouraged to call on the primary health care service for help... The AHA
should endeavour to provide night nurses if
necessary either from its own resources or,
for patients suffering from cancer, through
the Marie Curie Memorial Foundation's day and
night nursing service. The SSD might also, in
suitable circumstances, provide sitters from
its own night sitter service.

In discussing training for residential care
staff, it is observed that:

For instance some care staff might join
training programmes already being run by the
AHA for nursing auxiliaries. Staff of the
hospital departments of geriatric medicine and
psychiatry, as well as members of primary
health care teams... might be able to assist
in providing the instruction required...

Significant DHSS and professional reports

Under the heading of Administrative Nursing Advice it is stated that:

> ...it is anticipated that all professional nursing needed in residential Homes will eventually be provided by primary health care nurses employed by the AHA. Some health authorities may be hard pressed in attempting to stretch their nursing resources to cover entirely their statutory responsibility to the residents in local authority Homes... The provision of professional nursing facilities to local authority Homes should be regarded by AHAs as a high priority when planning the current deployment of nursing services.

11. PREVENTIVE MEDICINE, VOL.1, REPORT (First Report from the Expenditure Committee, 1977).

The DHSS and others, it was reported:

> approve of health visitors concerning themselves with old as well as with young; the Society of Community Medicine felt that people's inclination to seek medical advice from available "experts" who were not actually doctors, should be turned to account by using health visitors to advise the whole family. Our impression, from evidence given by the profession, is that informally they already do.
>   In evidence it was suggested by Dr E Steiner "that one benefit of the lower birthrate in Aberdeen was an improved service for the elderly by health visitors".

The committee felt that most health visitors still regarded their work with babies and young children as their first priority but:

> I find pressures on me to spend time visiting elderly people and I find that more of my time is taken up in clinical sessions, but since those clinical sessions are in the main devoted to the developmental examination of pre-school children it is perhaps a proper part of it. I regret the time I cannot spend in people's homes.

In discussing the fact that most health visitors are now attached to general practice, it was

Significant DHSS and professional reports

pointed out that this means that:

> the health visitor may no longer have a well-
> defined area to practise in so that she is no
> longer a well-known neighbourhood figure. This
> situation may be alleviated if a health visit-
> or works from a health centre within a well-
> defined geographical area, as the Sub-Commit-
> tee saw at Thamesmead.

Generally the sub-committee were much in favour of
health centres as the best way of accommodating and
promoting primary health care teams.
    The committee reported that:

> it was suggested by BUPA that nurses could
> carry out certain types of screening as eff-
> ectively as doctors and that other auxiliary
> staff could also be used more effectively. We
> understand from the FPA that there are schemes
> to use nurses to fit intra-uterine devices.

It was pointed out by Dr J J Murray that:

> speaking on behalf of the Royal College of
> Physicians, that the employment of auxiliary
> staff was not necessarily much cheaper than
> the employment of more highly trained people.

This was particularly where the auxiliary could
only practise with the fully trained person on
hand. This could lead to one or both of the fully
trained and auxiliary people being only partially
employed.
    The report suggests that certain routine
screening or checking should be undertaken by the
primary health care team:

> The Sub-Committee were told that it was very
> much cheaper to discover say 90% of cases of
> deafness in children by the use of health
> visitors than to detect 100% by the use of
> expensive specialists who had no other func-
> tions.

12. PREVENTION AND HEALTH (DHSS, DES, Scottish
Home and Health Department and Welsh Office, 1977).

    This white paper was the government's formal
response to the report of the Expenditure Committee
(1977) referred to above. It endorsed the role of

the primary health care team in preventive care. In addition to health visitors' crucial role in relation to babies and young children, the government also referred to their role (with district nurses) in preventive care of the elderly.

> Health visitors and district nurses can help with advice to the elderly about remaining active and about ways of safeguarding health. Many general practices have record systems which make it possible to identify elderly persons most at risk, for example, those living alone, the recently bereaved, those recently discharged from hospital and the over-75s. Members of the primary health care team can observe the environment as well as the general condition of individuals identified in this way; and it is possible, without the need for a formal screening service, to detect potential impairments which, if not corrected, could prove difficult to manage later on. Poor vision, impaired hearing, bad dentition, difficulty in walking, mental confusion, depression and incontinence need to be investigated and may require early referral to the appropriate service.

13. HEALTH SERVICES MANAGEMENT: THE EXTENDING ROLE OF THE CLINICAL NURSE - LEGAL IMPLICATIONS AND TRAINING REQUIREMENTS, Circular HC(77)22 (DHSS, 1977a).

In the letter accompanying this circular when issued, (CNO(77)9), the point is made that the role of the nurse was continually developing, and that nurses were constantly acquiring new skills to meet new needs. The working party which produced the circular HC(77)22 was aware that this extension could be in several ways, for example by development within the traditional nursing role, in response to an emergency and by delegation by doctors. However, it is where the nursing role is extended by delegation that there was felt to be a need for clarification and this explains the emphasis on this aspect in HC(77)22.

The circular took as its starting point the report of the Committee on Nursing (DHSS, Scottish Home and Health Department and Welsh Office, 1972). This report had considered the question of the overlapping functions of doctors and nurses. The circular HC(77)22 stated that this, the Briggs

Report, had emphasized the central differences between the caring role of nurses and the diagnostic
and curative functions of doctors. It had recognized that some of the differences and functions
were becoming less distinguishable and emphasized
the need for closer co-operation between the two
professions in the best interests of the patient.
The report had concluded that though there were no
apparent legal objections to continuing the existing practice of dividing work between the professions, nurses should be required to undertake only
those duties for which they had been educated and
trained.

As to legal implications, the circular
HC(77)22 states that :

> Work that had hitherto been carried out by
> doctors ought therefore to be delegated to
> nurses only when:
> a. the nurse has been specifically and ade-
>   quately trained for the performance of
>   the new task and she agrees to undertake
>   it;
> b. this training has been recognised as
>   satisfactory by the employing Authority;
> c. the new task has been recognised by the
>   professions and by the employing author-
>   ity as a task which may be properly dele-
>   gated to a nurse;
> d. the delegating doctor has been assured of
>   the competence of the individual nurse
>   concerned.

Health authorities were asked to review areas
where delegation to nurses would be desirable. The
importance was stressed of health authorities having a clearly defined policy based on prior local
discussion and agreement between those responsible
for providing nursing and medical facilities and
made known in writing to all staff who were likely
to be involved. In particular the policy should
specify:

> a. what tasks may be delegated;
> b. what qualifications and training are
>   necessary before a nurse may accept
>   particular delegated tasks, and
> c. what safeguards must accompany the dele-
>   gation of particular tasks in order that
>   the safety of the patient is not jeopard-
>   ized.

14. AN INVESTIGATION INTO THE PRINCIPLES OF HEALTH VISITING (CETHV, 1977).

This was a report produced by a working party set up by the Council for the Education and Training of Health Visitors 'to examine the principles and practice of health visiting' as a pre-requisite to revision of the training curriculum.

In order to formulate new principles it was necessary to have an agreed definition of health visiting viz:

The professional practice of health visiting consists of planned activities aimed at the promotion of health and prevention of ill health. It thereby contributes substantially to individual and social well being by focusing attention at various times on either an individual, a social group or a community. It has three unique functions:

i. identifying and fulfilling self declared and recognised as well as unacknowledged and unrecognised, health needs of individuals and social groups;

ii. providing a generalist health agent service in an era of increasing specialisation in the health care available to individuals and communities;

iii. monitoring simultaneously the health needs and demands of individuals and communities, contributing to the fulfilment of these needs, and facilitating appropriate care and service by other professional health care groups.

The principles formulated by the working party were:

i. The search for health needs

ii. The stimulation of the awareness of health needs

iii. The influence on policies affecting health

iv. The facilitation of health-enhancing activities.

The remainder of the publication was mostly taken up with a discussion of the principles and, amongst others, the following points were made.

The search for health needs

In discussing how to make search effective, the importance of a scientific approach to the making of observations, interpretations and deductions from data was stressed and of the need to validate conclusions by collecting new facts to refute or confirm early hypotheses. The working party thought that it was 'therefore, imperative to devise tools of evaluation in health visiting'.

It was argued, however, that it is not enough to rely on the scientific method or at least a narrow interpretation of that method given the nature of human beings. It was also noted that:

> Less random and more effective health visiting could be practised by visiting at non-critical points in the life-cycle [something it was pointed out that health visitors have always recognized for identifying certain health needs]. However, just as the concept of selective screening has fallen into disrepute because it proved impossible to ensure the normality of the excluded "normal" group, so the concept of vulnerable periods in the life span has yet to be tested rigorously.

Stimulation of an awareness of health needs

After an analysis of the meaning of need, the following points amongst others were made:

> To encourage and stimulate an awareness of health needs, to motivate individuals and families to improve their own conditions, to take community action for better housing, schools, play areas and health services by teaching the value of health, must be a priority of health visitors and others.
>
> ...The Sheffield study on Sudden Infant Deaths has shown the effective contribution, in an area of previously unmet need, which can be made by an adequate number of health visiting staff co-ordinated so as to concentrate on a specific group.
>
> ...the prevention of mental illness by health teaching on psychosocial needs from infancy, should be one of the health visitor's main priorities.
>
> ...It may follow that aspects of need which cannot be dealt with immediately might well be fulfilled in the longer term, once they are uncovered and recognised; for ex-

ample, where no nursery education is available, the health visitor could co-operate with parents in establishing play groups.
In the past it may not have been a deliberate feature of health visiting practice to engage in participative activity with the community but a new partnership approach will be needed.
...The health visiting profession has a responsibility for the health of the whole population. This claim is idealistic at a time when the number of health visitors is in such a poor proportion to the population...'

The working party felt that it was very important to continue with normal routine visiting of families by health visitors.

The influence on policies affecting health
If it is accepted that health is of value and worthy of achievement, then the health visiting profession has a responsibility to influence policies that affect health and in order to achieve this, health visitors will have to engage in political activity.
...The full implications of this principle [namely the influence on policies affecting health] then, are that health visitors seek to exert an influence on policies affecting people's health and that in applying this principle they will engage in political activity designed to support policies conducive to health and to challenge policies not conducive to health.
...For the purpose of any further elaboration of this principle it is important to distinguish the three levels at which health visitors seek to influence policies affecting health. The national or macroscopic level is illustrated in the activities of the professional body collectively; the individual or microscopic level is illustrated in the activities of individual health visitors acting with or upon other individuals and families; finally the intermediate mediascopic level, is illustrated in the activities of one or a group of health visitors acting at local or community level.

Significant DHSS and professional reports

Examples of activities at the various levels are
given and among other points made are:

> ...it is more than likely that in their daily
> work individual health visitors seek to inf-
> luence courses of action relevant to people's
> health either planned or carried out by local
> government departments, for example the Social
> Services Department, the Housing Department or
> the Education Department. They may seek to
> influence the Electricity Board or the Water
> Board. They may be acting on behalf of one
> particular individual or family or they may be
> acting on behalf of many...

The importance of health visitors being part of the
primary health care team was stressed particularly
as it was pointed out that the work of the health
visitor was often not fully understood by general
practitioners and the role of the health visitor in
influencing policies was seen within the primary
health care team too.

> The health visitor might wish to influ-
> ence GPs policy on behalf of one of his pat-
> ients either by supporting it or challenging
> it.
> ...At the local community level their
> [that is the health visitors] contributions to
> social change can be seen in their encourage-
> ment of interaction between groups of parents
> with similar needs. In this way they are
> instrumental in the creation of action groups
> which in turn provide facilities such as play
> groups and toy libraries for children, day
> centres for the elderly or any other health
> facility for which there is a local need.
> They are also concerned about the adverse
> effects upon children living in high-rise
> buildings or in other housing conditions which
> are detrimental to health...

The facilitation of health-enhancing activities
> ...The "facilitation" or "enabling" aspect of
> health visitors will be seen to operate at two
> distinct levels. First, at the client level
> where the health visitor seeks to facilitate
> some activity or behaviour desired in or by
> the client. This is normally achieved through
> counselling or health teaching activities.
> Second, at the colleague level where the

> intention is to facilitate activity within the
> health team (or related teams), for the bene-
> fit of the client or the client group. This
> latter intention may be achieved through com-
> munication and referral within the team so as
> to initiate planned activity on behalf of the
> client.

It was pointed out that the concept of the health
visitor as a facilitator was not new and certainly
dated back to the Jameson Report (Ministry of
Health, 1956) and subsequently supported by other
professional pronouncements.

In the concluding chapter of the book further
issues are discussed in the course of which the
following points were made:

> The question is often asked "what is
> unique about health visitors?" The answer is
> that it lies in the combination of their spec-
> ific areas of knowledge and particular skills
> which is unique; and that they are the only
> professional workers to visit "normal" fam-
> ilies with a view to the promotion of health
> and prevention of illness...
> ...One particular dilemma in relation to
> practice that seems to concern practitioners,
> which is again ultimately related to princ-
> iples is "are we or are we not practitioners
> in our own right?" Perhaps Donald Hicks has
> already answered this once and for all by
> suggesting that none of us is. Health visit-
> ors are salaried employees of a statutory body
> and in this respect cannot possibly be pract-
> itioners in their own right. The pamphlet
> "The Function of the Health Visitor" (CETHV,
> 1967) offers an explanation by saying that
> health visitors detect cases of need on
> personal initiative as well as acting upon
> referrals. Even if they ever were, health
> visitors are no longer free agents with regard
> to detection and action for they operate
> within powerful constraints, not least of
> which are the expectations others have of the
> role of the health visitor.
> The statement could also mean that health
> visitors are free to exercise their own judge-
> ments within their recognised spheres of act-
> ivity and will accept responsibility for so
> doing... Perhaps this particular dilemma is

related to influencing policies at the micro level, "will someone give me the authority to challenge those policies of colleagues in other professions which in my considered judgement are not in the best interests of my client?" It should not be necessary to make this plea since health visitors are members of primary health care teams and teamwork should imply agreed courses of action.

Another dilemma of practice related to the above seems to be the "attachment" controversy. It would appear ... that many health visitors feel they were more effective when they were operating in geographically defined areas. This may or may not be so since "effectiveness" in health visiting is difficult to define, but irrespective of proof attachment and effectiveness obviously pose problems.

This publication was designed to stimulate discussion and a good deal of debate took place within the profession following the release of this report, some of which was published in 'The Investigation Debate - A Commentary on an Investigation into the Principles of Health Visiting' (CETHV, 1980).

Among the points made which were particularly relevant to this book were the following:

The report exhorts a continuing appraisal of the basis of health visiting - with due respect I suggest we should consider another appraisal - that of the needs of the community. What do the public need? Do they need home visits, advice, nursing care, medical care? ... What are the expectations of the public and how can we meet them, seems a more sound basis for an investigation than principles on which academic training is based.

(This was part of a paper given by Miss D Blenkinsop at the conference held in Durham, October 1978 when she was referring in particular to the fourth principle, 'the facilitation of health-enhancing activities'.)

Points arising from conference discussion groups included the following (in respect of 'Aspects Relating to the Community'):

However it is also evident that many of the public are not aware of the aims and scope of health visitors' work. Linked with this were frequent suggestions that public relations and marketing techniques should be used to sell health and health visiting.

In the context of the 'Availability of Service', a number of factors affecting availability of services were mentioned, including:

staffing levels, the provision of complementary and ancillary services, and area policy affecting the availability of the health visiting service. The physical aspects of premises as well as their location relative to residential or central shopping areas were also considered to be important.

Availability of services can also be affected by the extent to which referrals made to the service are appropriate and by individual differences in practitioners' interpretation of the health visitor role and function (such as personal preferences for particular kinds of work or age groups):

These individual differences interact with the area health profiles and policies, sizes of caseload, provision of complementary services which in turn affect the availability of the health visitor. Since the health visitor sees herself as a practitioner in her own right (within a multi-professional service) conflict often arises when her selection of priority differs from management. The level at which decision-making is allowed, also varies from area to area leading to management /field dissension.

Other points at issue included regular routine visiting versus crisis visiting; the growth of telephone consultation as a replacement for home visiting; the felt need for a 24-hour service to be available to the public. It was stated that the health visiting service has not been sufficiently flexible in meeting changes in the public's working hours, particularly with the increasing number of working mothers.

In the context of 'Programming of Service', the following point was made:

The question of generalist or specialist health visitors was raised. Some health visitors want to develop skills in particular applications of health visiting (eg. to the severely mentally or physically handicapped, geriatric care in the community, specialised health teaching), and may have specific aptitudes. Research is required to assess which method gives the best service to families with special needs.

In the context of 'The Base for Practice', among the points made were the following:

It was argued by some that a selective return to geographical areas would have many advantages, particularly where a high density population exists or where there is a continuously moving population eg. high rise flats and decaying inner cities. For those health visitors who operate in multi-GP areas or in areas in which zoning takes place, a geographically based service would reduce both travelling time and expenses, as well as reduce the possibilities for those who fail to make use of health services, to slip through the net.
On the other hand, the very nature and composition of attachment alerts both the public and other professional staff to the inclusion of the health visitor in health caring activities. However it was stated that no research evidence exists to support the view that GP attachment increases the public's use of the health visitor service. It was felt by many that GP attachment provides for access to and utilisation of more information, as well as contributing to the means of developing better communication between those who make decisions about patient or family treatment and provision.
Others felt that a geographical basis for practice helped the public to identify the responsible health visitor. The point was made that there was no evidence about the effect on the use of the health visitor service, of basing health visitors centrally in a health centre or in more dispersed locations.

In the context of the 'Evaluation of Service', the following was said:

It was argued by many that efforts must
be made to determine the criteria for the
evaluation of practice in terms of agreed general and specific objectives. Until this had
been accomplished, it would be difficult to
evaluate the cost-effectiveness of the
service.
It was suggested that it should be possible to compare the effectiveness and cost of
geographically-based and GP-attached health
visiting; different referral systems; the effectiveness of home visiting; the effect on infant mortality and morbidity of differing
health visitor population ratios. Many health
visitors wished to see more research into
practice, especially by health visitors.

15. A HAPPIER OLD AGE - A DISCUSSION DOCUMENT ON
ELDERLY PEOPLE IN OUR SOCIETY (DHSS, Welsh Office,
1978).

This document had the following to say about
community nurses:

At present, just under 50% of cases dealt with
by district nurses and about 15% of those of
health visitors involve elderly people. Both
the health visiting and district nursing services have responsibilities to other priority
groups such as young children and it can be
argued that health visitors should spend proportionately less time with elderly people and
district nurses proportionately more. Nursing
auxiliaries, with suitable supervision and in-
service training, can often provide the kind
of care needed by many elderly people. Personal tasks that many elderly people find
difficult include bathing and cutting toe
nails.

The report asked:

What is the scope for adjusting the roles of
community nurses and for expanding the help
provided by auxiliary staff within the district nursing service?

Significant DHSS and professional reports

16. COLLABORATION IN COMMUNITY CARE - A DISCUSSION
DOCUMENT (Central Health Services Council and the
Personal Social Services Council, 1978).

This is the report of a working party set up
by the Central Health Services Council and the
Personal Social Services Council. It is predominantly concerned with relationships between the
social services on the one hand and general practitioners and health authorities on the other hand;
but there are some references to community nurses
in the field and some observations about the nature
of teamwork.
In speaking of the primary health care team,
the report refers to a confusion between the roles
of health visitor and social worker and some overlap, and more generally points to the fact that
problems of collaboration could be partly overcome
if health and social services staff, particularly
those in charge, were better informed about each
other. The report goes on to say that one of the
ways that such knowledge could be obtained would be
through inter-personal exchanges during training
both before and after qualifying. Shared training
between nursing and social work should be encouraged, in particular between health visitors and
social workers.
By attachment, the report means:

an arrangement whereby a member of one profession has a formalized means of working with
another professional group within the latter's
own territory.

Note that this definition of attachment allows various degrees of attachment, with the attached member of staff working within the other professional's territory for any time between a half day
a week, and a whole week with freedom in the former
case to deal with other clients on another basis.
In referring to schemes of attachment for
health authority personnel to social service departments, the following examples were cited as
arising from the survey which was undertaken in
connection with this report:

a district nurse attached to a day centre,
district nurse seconded to a home for the
elderly... and attachment of a health visitor
to a day nursery and play group.

17. REPORT (Royal Commission on the National Health Service, 1979).

The report drew attention to the shortage of nurses working in the community which placed a strain on them and 'reduced the effectiveness of other members of the primary care teams'. Whilst supporting the concept of attachment for community nurses, the report argued that there was a need for the health visitor to have an 'identifiable geographical area for case finding'. It was also mentioned that where the general practitioner's list is widely dispersed, this may mean additional travelling for attached district nurses compared with the situation where they were responsible for a geographical patch. Mention was made of the possible conflict of loyalties of the attached community nurse between the primary care team of which she was a part and her superiors in nursing management.

In examining the possibility of extending the role of nurses in primary care, it was stated that 'the role of the midwife may serve as a model of the extended role and clinical responsibilities which nurses could carry'. It was noted that 'the midwife makes her own judgements about the supervision, care and advice to women before and after childbirth' and that in 75% of deliveries, according to the Royal College of Midwives, the midwife was the senior person present. It was also pointed out that nurses working in the community 'have long had a considerable degree of independence'.

The Commission thought 'it is possible that district nurses could undertake more first visits to patients in their home' (quoting the experiment carried out at the Woodside Health Centre in Glasgow, Moore et al. 1973). It was pointed out that in North America

> nurse practitioners have proved to be perfectly acceptable to patients, and indeed are often felt to be more accessible than the doctor, particularly as in the main they operate in under-doctored areas.

The Commission drew attention to the finding of MacGuire (1977) that:

> the involvement of nurses in screening both the very young and the elderly is already well accepted ... it is not yet routine in all

practice settings for nurses to be the main contact with elderly patients. ... In many cases the nurses are effectively making first contact decisions anyway though this may not always be recognised for what it is.

More generally, the Royal Commission endorsed the view of regional nursing officers in England that:

Examination should be given to the possibility of extending the role of the nurse and enabling them to undertake tasks traditionally the province of the medical staff. ...There is a need in some long-stay care areas for nurses to take the lead. Nurses should be enabled and encouraged to prescribe nursing care programmes including the mobilisation of other services such as physiotherapy and occupational therapy.

It was felt that any move towards extending the role of the nurse should not be at the expense of their caring function, and also the Commission reported the concern of the Royal College of Nursing about some extensions of the role of the nurse in respect of the legal liability of nurses involved and their ability to cope in relation to their training.
It was considered:

There are increasingly important roles for community nurses, not just in the treatment room but in health surveillance for vulnerable groups and in screening procedures, health education and preventive programmes, and as a point of first contact, particularly for the young and the elderly.

Research was recommended into the following aspects of the work of community nurses:

the workload of district nursing and the respective demands of domiciliary care and treatment room work;
the respective roles of district nurse, treatment room nurse and practice nurse vis-a-vis the general practitioner;
the use of aides in community nursing;
and standards of care.

18. THE EXTENDED CLINICAL ROLE OF THE NURSE (Royal College of Nursing of the United Kingdom, 1979).

This guidance to members in effect endorsed that of the DHSS Health Circular HC(77)22, 'The Extending Role of the Clinical Nurse - Legal Implications and Training Requirements', (see page 56) in the limited area with which that was concerned (that is the delegation to nurses of tasks hitherto regarded as being in the field of work of the doctor). It did, however, seek to take a rather wider view free from concentration on identification of specific tasks which constitute the extension or development of the clinical nursing role. Indeed the RCN considered that it should not provide lists of examples of the extended role, but that the matter should be discussed in general philosphical terms. 'Lists are, by nature, limiting.'

'It was considered that as nursing was an independent profession, the independent practitioner should have the freedom to plan care.' In searching for an appropriate definition of the word 'care' it was suggested that

nursing care means meeting the individual patient's self-care potential in all dimensions of his activities of daily living without usurping the patient's/client's own role ... Nurses should establish their own parameters of care and then discuss them with the medical and remedial professions.
...Clinical nurses have tended to look to others for guidance and direction rather than making their own decisions about planning and developing care.

But some nurses are ready to develop a more independent approach given the autonomy to do so.

The profession has the responsibility to see that they are encouraged and not inhibited safeguarding, at the same time, against a decline in essential nursing care. [The rights of nurses who do not wish to extend their role to include a greater degree of autonomy of practice are also to be 'recognised and respected'.] ...the autonomy of the nurse must involve an extension of her professional managerial discretion in relation to the doctor and her superiors.

Greater autonomy will involve some eman-
cipation from controls by both the medical
treatment system and from the hierarchy within
nursing. However, the development of a management nursing system which allows clinical
autonomy is equally an issue of management
strategy. One of the major problem areas
seems to be the formulation and implementation
of nursing policy. This can produce constraints on the clinical nurse in that it can
have a restrictive effect on clinical practice. In order to minimise these constraints a
more effective working relationship needs to
be established between senior nurse managers
and clinical practitioners.

19. PRIMARY HEALTH CARE NURSING - A TEAM APPROACH.
Report of a working party (Royal College of Nursing, Society of Primary Health Care Nursing,1980).

This working party was set up to produce a
document setting out the independent and inter-
dependent role of primary care nurses in this
country. The term 'nurse' was used in this report
as a generic term to include district nurse and
health visitor (and midwife, but we shall not consider her role). The report considered the role
and functions of the various primary care nurses,
noting that there are areas of overlap in these
roles. Thus for example, it is within the competence of the health visitor and the district nurse
to provide certain advice to patients and their
families.
Accordingly in their discussion of the inter-
dependent roles of primary care nurses, two points
are made. First of all knowledge, not only of the
formal disciplinary capabilities of team members,
but also of the particular interests of team members is important. If there is this knowledge,
then appropriate people can be brought in to give
care; 'appropriate' being used in a way that partly
transcends disciplinary boundaries. Secondly the
point is made that the question of who does what as
for example between the district nurse and the
health visitor, or between the district nurse and a
doctor, depends in part on context. Thus for example, if a procedure like an injection is needed
in the case of a patient already being visited by a
district nurse, then provided that this was within
her competence she should do it. If on the other
hand there is not this particular established cont-

act, then it makes sense for the doctor not to delegate it but to do it him/herself at the time when it is recommended. It is observed that there are considerable advantages in this approach to the patient. They receive a service from whichever member of the team can best help them at that time. There are no duplicated visits, they are being cared for by a united group who work together in their best interests.

In discussing future developments of primary care nursing, several difficulties are mentioned which may prevent the nursing members of the team from attaining the role, both independent and inter-dependent, described in the earlier part of the report. One of these is the absence of attachment or other suitable links with general practitioners. If the district nursing and health visiting services operate on a geographical basis, and if the geographic areas are conterminous, it is still possible for there to be a team approach between these two services.

Another difficulty may be the proliferation of specialist nurses (as distinct from general workers within the primary health care team who develop a special interest, for example in the problems of adolescence). The working party was not 'in principle, opposed to the development of specialist nurses...'. It may be that specialist nurses

> provide the kind of nursing skill which, either because it is based on training in a different specialty or because it is rarely required, cannot appropriately be acquired by all district nurses. On the other hand specialist nurses may be used to give a type of care which it should be possible for every district nursing team to give

provided the caseload is not too large. This could take the interest out of district nursing, the working party observed. They also noted the development of specialist health visitor posts, for example for the handicapped and elderly where the same problem would arise. With each development of an additional group of specialist nurses, it was thought, another area of work, often a challenging area, would be lost to the ordinary primary health care staff.

Two points are made on the professional aspects of the primary health care nurses' work. Because in certain circumstances an employer can be held responsible for the acts of an employee, employers are able to specify the range of duties which may be performed by their staff. Given an increasing tendency to resort to litigation, this had led employing authorities to restrict the duties that may be carried out to a point at which staff (usually nurses) are unable to fulfil their role, or to exercise their professional judgement. An example of this is that community nurses have always suggested 'over the counter' remedies for common complaints, but some health authorities have been suggesting that they should stop doing this. The working party argues that nurses should continue doing this and take the consequences if they are at fault in their judgement, as ordinary accountable professionals.

The second point made is that restrictions are sometimes placed on activities for nursing members of the primary health care team, because of an imperfect appreciation of their role and functions by their superiors. This is more likely to occur when those managing services have little or no experience of the work involved. When these posts are held by those who do have such experience, it appears more likely that community nurses will receive support and guidance.

Health visitor training should equip the health visitor to define health care goals and subsequently to evaluate the effectiveness of the work. It is to be hoped that health care consumers will increasingly be involved in both the planning and evaluation of the health visiting services.

Two factors will continue to affect the kind of work undertaken in the future by district nurses. The first is that the demographic changes which have been predicted, may result in an increase in the number of patients with degenerative conditions requiring nursing care. The second is that as the period of post-operative care in hospitals becomes shorter, the amount of support and care required from community based staff will increase. This will require an efficient and effective system of communication between the district and hospital sister.

Finally the point is made that expanding or extending the role of the nurse can take place in two ways; firstly by a widening of the role to take over tasks formerly undertaken by other disciplines and secondly by increasing the depth of the approach to the problems, that is to say giving very comprehensive care to one patient or client in a more or less traditional nursing sense, 'seeing that person as an individual in a specific family and community' and discovering 'health needs and problems beyond those which are immediately obvious'. Possibly, the report concludes,

> both a broadening and a deepening of roles is required, but breadth should not be achieved at the cost of depth.

20. CARE IN ACTION. A HANDBOOK OF POLICIES AND PRIORITIES FOR THE HEALTH AND PERSONAL SOCIAL SERVICES IN ENGLAND (DHSS, 1981).

This 'Handbook of Policies and Priorities for the Health and Personal Social Services in England' produced under a Conservative government reaffirmed government support (see pages 47 and 50 above) for a strong primary health care service. This service was to include early detection of illness, swifter treatment to prevent deterioration, care of people in the community rather than in hospital and drawing on the resources of the family, neighbours and voluntary groups rather than over-reliance on the services of full-time professionals in hospitals. In particular it stated that more health visitors and district nurses were needed in many places and that authorities should aim to increase secondments for training. In an appendix under the heading 'Early discharge schemes, day surgery and other developments', it stated that there was some evidence that more district nursing functions might be performed by less highly qualified members of the team and also that there may be some overlap between the services provided by the district nurse team (particularly the nurse auxiliaries) and the home helps provided by social services departments. It suggested that these issues raised questions which merited further studies about the organization and operation of the district nursing team and the lack of relationship between these teams and home help services.

21. HEALTH VISITING IN THE 80s. (Health Visitors' Association, 1981).

This document is a revised edition of 'Health Visiting in the Seventies' (Health Visitors' Association, 1975) and states that:

the biggest challenge to the concentration of health visiting on its traditional function of caring for mothers and young children has come from the development generally known as "attachment" to general practitioners.

One of the problems encountered in attachment schemes, was that:

Too few general practitioners understood the independent responsibilities of the health visitor. She is thought to be useful for routine visiting of elderly patients, answering calls and selecting the doctors' visits, giving immunisation injections and coping with over-persistent surgery attenders and she may be considered unco-operative if unwilling to fulfil these functions.

The other main arguments of those who question the wisdom of attachment for health visiting, concern the effect on the service given by the health visitors and the cost of providing those services:

It is contended that some of the people most in need of advice and support from health visitors tend to move frequently and do not register with the general practitioner at all unless they become ill, that the health visitor's attention is likely to be directed away from those most vulnerable, and hence most in need, to those who make themselves most noticeable in the doctor's surgery and that a health visitor regularly visiting in the same geographical area becomes a well-known figure easily approachable, for example, by a newly arrived young mother or neighbours worried about the well-being of a child, who will not know where to turn if different health visitors make only rare appearances visiting their own "practice patients". Furthermore, development of attachment arrangements tends towards disappearance of the conveniently situated local clinic where health visitors are known to be readily available to all who need them and the doctor's surgery or even a new health centre will probably be both less conveniently situated and less welcoming.
The cost of providing health visitors' services when each has to call at homes over a more widely scattered area and two or more may

well be visiting in the same road, block, or
even house, is inevitably greater than when
each one restricts her visiting to a prescribed section of the map.

On the other hand, arguments in support of
attachment are that

all members of the primary health care team
benefit from regular contact with each other
and hence are able to provide a better overall
service to the public with the avoidance of
any conflicting advice, and the advantage of
discussion of problems and that it provides an
opportunity for health visitors to interest
general practitioners in preventive medicine.
...Some, if not all, the arguments against the attachment of health visitors to general practices would clearly disappear if
practice lists were restricted to defined geographic areas, all general practitioners were
tidily grouped into conveniently situated
local health centres and there were enough
health visitors to go round. In the meantime,
however, the Health Visitors' Association suggests that a great deal more careful study is
required before the setting of all health visiting within primary health care teams can be
fully confirmed as beneficial for the people
for whom the service is designed and maintained.

Health visitors are now also 'part of a vast
hierarchical structure of nursing management'.
However, since

the integration of the health services on the
1st April 1974, and in the new nursing management structure, despite vigorous protestation
and regular representations by the Health Visitors' Association, it is quite possible for a
health visitor to find that no one above her
has any experience of health visiting at all
and quite probably that only the Nursing Officer will have health visiting experience and
no one above middle management (Senior Nursing
Officer) will have had any experience in any
of the community services.

The paper then goes on to list the functions of health visitors, classified according to three levels of priority:

1. **Recommended selection of work for health visitors working within severe staff shortages.**
   Urgent home visiting, i.e. to new births; to newly arrived families with small children; actual or suspected cases of non-accidental injury to children; in response to requests from families; to handicapped children; to newly-reported TB cases; to ante-natal mothers, especially primiparae.
   Urgent referrals from other agencies which are properly within the health visitor's province.
   Efficient record-keeping.
   Involvement in the training of student health visitors.
   Child Health Clinics.

2. **Recommended additional work for health visitors working under only average pressure.**
   Routine visiting of all children up to school age.
   Visits to all ante-natal mothers.
   Supportive visits to families under temporary stress.
   Follow-up of immunization failures.
   Paediatric developmental testing at home of non-clinic attenders.
   Health teaching to groups of adults and in schools.
   Further liaison with hospitals and proffessional colleagues.
   Involvement in the training of medical students, student nurses and social work students.

3. **Recommended additions for health visitors who may, one day, have really small case-loads.**
   Routine visiting of all children up to school-leaving age with time to attend to the needs of all members of the family.
   Support for families under stress from e.g. psychiatric problems, chronic illness, handicap.
   Counselling and health education at family planning and cytology sessions and

other appropriate clinics.
Visits to play groups and nurseries.
Involvement in research projects.
Regular visits to schools and hospital wards.

22. PRIMARY HEALTH CARE IN EUROPE. THE ROLE OF THE HEALTH VISITOR. Report of a Conference held July 1981 (Wilson (Ed.), 1981).

The conference was attended by 140 health visitors/public health nurses from 15 countries in Europe and was jointly organized by the Council for the Education and Training of Health Visitors, the Health Visitors' Association, the Royal College of Nursing, the National Standing Conference of Representatives of Health Visitor Education and Training Centres (UK), North East London Polytechnic and the World Health Organization (Regional Office for Europe).
It was thought that this conference was the first meeting concerned with primary health care to be organized by health visitors/public health nurses in the European region.
The thinking of conference delegates was summed up in the final group report prepared by Charlotte Kratz and Gabrielle Markes, some brief extracts from which are quoted below:

Moving Towards Primary Health Care
... the idea of health visitors/public health nurses deciding their priorities and in community involvement by health visitors/public health nurses, rather than continuing to provide one to one services to which health visitors in the U.K. were used

was discussed, given the shortage of resources.

The client should be paramount in all decisions pertaining to his own health care.
...One major obstacle to moving towards primary health care is the growth of specialist services which in many cases take over the work of health visitors. This is undesirable in every way. While specialist advice should be readily available specialists should not take over from existing general services. The example of France, where the variety of specialist services were such that people did not know any longer whom to consult loomed large.

The Role of the Health Visitor/Public Health Nurse Today

...The role should change to meet the needs of the community which the health service served.

...The care of mothers and young children seemed to be a universal charge on health visitors. There was discussion on whether it was more appropriate for health visitors to respond to all calls made on them, possibly at the expense of the quality of their care, or to concentrate on only a few groups.

Participants were in no doubt that health visitors/public health nurses in primary care should be generalists, though in countries at present separating the preventive and curative function this separation should be maintained. They should be able to call on the services of specialists but should at all times be able to maintain control.

The difficulties of working in primary health care and other teams were spelled out. Nevertheless it was considered appropriate that health visitors should continue to function in such teams.

The Influence of the Environment on the Work of Health Visitors/Public Health Nurses

The influence of politics on nursing was a paramount theme throughout the week. Politics were seen as being party politics, pressure group politics, or professional politics, and in all these nurses should be involved...

...the influence of the geographical environment and of the immediate environment such as living in urban or rural areas was talked about. All these affected the work situation, e.g. the need for a triple duty worker rather than three individuals.

The Relationship between Education and Practice in Health Visiting/Public health Nursing

There was much commendation of the "Principles of Health Visiting" [see summary on page 58 of this chapter] which people felt were universally applicable.

Nursing process was seen as a suitable systematic model for teaching health visiting.

...If health visitors are to be prepared to give a suitable and sensitive service to clients, then management had a responsibility to see that appropriate support for them was available.

The Way Forward
There was an urgent need to use existing research findings and to commission further research, particularly by nurses. There was a plea for just distribution of available research monies.

Clients and communities should be involved in evaluating the services available to them and the people providing the service.

23. THE PRIMARY HEALTH CARE TEAM - REPORT OF A JOINT WORKING GROUP (Standing Medical Advisory Committee and The Standing Nursing and Midwifery Advisory Committee, 1981). (The Harding Committee).

The terms of reference of this committee were 'to examine problems associated with the establishment and operation of primary health care teams and to recommend solutions'. In its introduction, the report stated that the committee was set up because of a 'growing awareness that in some areas belief in the concept of the primary health care team was waning'. And indeed, in a number of areas particularly in inner city areas, nurse attachment arrangements had been or were being dismantled because of problems of providing adequate nursing care to the community as a whole, or for reasons of economy. The committee did find evidence of waning support for the attachment of community nurses to general practitioners. Among the reasons for this were diseconomies of attachment as compared with giving a nurse a geographical patch, which became exacerbated when there was a shortage of community nurses in that locality necessitating re-deployment often at short notice from one practice to another. There were felt to be actual losses in departing from the geographical patch approach in that the nurse found it more difficult to be familiar with her clientele in the circumstances in which they lived when working with a doctor's list as distinct from the population within a defined geographical patch. In certain areas such as those in inner cities, a number of patients were not on the lists of doctors and so failed to receive community nursing services. It was stated that in one area, one seventh of the children below the age of five were not being visited by health visitors for this reason. Inadequate or unsuitable premises are another reason why attachment was disliked by some nursing authorities at least in that it reduced the possibility of effective teamwork. There was also a mention of problems in relationships between general practitioners and nursing officers in the community nursing services.

In particular there was sometimes difficulty arising out of conflict between health authority policy and the general practitioner's expectations of what a nurse should do, for example in the fields of vaccination, immunization and of family planning. Another difficulty was the way in which attached nurses were swopped around to cover the sickness or holidays of colleagues with the minimum of consultation with general practitioners.

In its conclusions and recommendations, the committee continued to endorse attachment of community nursing staff to general practices as probably the best way of promoting primary health care teamwork but recommended the zoning of group practice areas, particularly in inner city areas, but also in rural areas, so as to make it easier for community nurses to operate more or less on a geographical patch basis.

Among more specific recommendations were the following:

> Research should be conducted into levels of patient dependence on nursing services in the community in relation to the various levels of nursing skills and experience available in primary health care teams [that is the mix of trained support staff within nursing teams from the community].

That the relevant organizations

> should consider the role of the practice nurse, her relationship with health authority employed nurses and her need for training.
> ...constraints which place limits on the range of duties which health authority employed nurses may undertake should be subject to periodic review by health authorities in consultation with local medical committees along with any other factors which might prevent attached nursing staff working alongside general practitioners in surgery based treat-

ment rooms.
...Health authorities should, as soon as
possible, make arrangements to provide night
and weekend nursing services where these are
not already in existence.

24. PRIMARY HEALTH CARE IN INNER LONDON - Report
of a study group. (London Health Planning Consortium, 1981). (The Acheson Report).

This group, reporting at the same time as the
Harding Committee, broadly speaking endorsed the
findings in the Harding Committee's Report (see
page 80) but elaborated on a number of issues specific to primary health care in inner London.
They raised a number of issues concerned with
the problem of role definition and responsibilities
in primary health care. They noted that managers
of the community nursing and social work services
claim that general practitioners often fail to com-
prehend fully or sympathize with the extent of
their responsibilities to the population as a
whole. They recommended that 'health authorities
and local authorities should as far as possible
adopt common areas for which groups of primary care
workers were responsible and co-operate in the
joint provision of premises'. It was felt that
there was 'insufficient information relating to the
full extent and effect of the overlap of GP practices in densely populated inner city areas', and
recommended 'that priority should be given to spon-
soring research in this field'. Whilst recognizing
the fundamental principle that patients should be
able to choose their GP, the arrangement they favoured was one in which 'a group practice would be
teamed with a group of nurses and other primary
care workers' working as far as possible from the
same premises, providing services for the same
population. It was recognized that this could not
be achieved universally, however it was recommended
that
LMCs and FPCs in consultation with the
appropriate authorities should encourage
groups of GPs to concentrate their practice
areas so as to facilitate close working relationships with other primary care workers.
The health and local authorities should as a
matter of priority, ensure the organisation of
the working areas of other members of the
primary care team parallel to those of the
GPs.

...[Such practice areas] could be divided geographically to allow a "patch" responsibility for the other primary care workers. It would then be possible to identify people within the practice area who were not registered with the GPs but who nevertheless were entitled to and needed health care.

Turning to various types of nurse working in primary health care, they noted the prevalence of practice employed nurses in England (although they were not so common in London). They could see the advantage of the practice nurse to the GP in that it enabled the GP to make the best use of his/her own skills and 'she can also perform tasks under his supervision which health authorities · are unwilling to authorize their nurses to perform'. However, they also accepted that there was a view that the employment of nurses by GPs 'is not in the best interest of the professional management, training and development of those concerned'. The committee 'decided to make no recommendations which would disturb the present balance between community and practice nurses'.
Turning to the 'wider problem of role definition in primary health care', the report states:

With a large group of professionals operating in the same area there is bound to be an overlap of responsibilities and scope for changing the boundaries between different professions. Even within a single profession there are areas of concern. What for instance, is the appropriate balance and proportion of staffing between SENs and SRNs in district nursing? But there is also the much wider question of whether the total resources could be better used if the roles of different professions were less rigidly defined. There has been considerable discussion of the development of nurse practitioners who might, with appropriate training, take on some of the first point of contact work leaving the GP free to concentrate on the more complex medical questions. There are almost certainly overlaps between the roles of the health visitor and social worker and the boundaries between their work and that of general practitioners are not precise. It is also being suggested that there is scope for the development of care assistants to provide a combination of social, domestic and nursing care in order to maintain in the community patients who otherwise would have to be admitted to hospital - more for social than medical reasons. We RECOMMEND, however, that the DHSS should institute a review of the existing research on profesional roles in primary health care and consider whether further study is needed.

Another recommendation of the Acheson Report was:

that an experiment should be established in one of the health districts with a particularly high percentage of elderly living alone to "screen" on a regular basis all those over the age of 75. It is not envisaged that this should necessarily involve medical "screening" in the fullest sense of the word.... Rather it would be a service run under the supervision of community nurses - although not necessarily by them - to keep a watch on the general health and well-being of the elderly in the district, especially those living alone with no immediate family support. An important aim of such a project would be to identify the real costs of the service and whether screening by ensuring earlier detection and treatment might enable compensating savings to be made in direct services.

The committee recommended that where child attendance rates at accident and emergency departments are sufficiently high, the appointment of liaison health visitors to these departments should be considered and that in any event where children attend accident and emergency departments, a note of their attendance should be sent to their health visitor as well as to the general practitioner.

25. THE ROLE OF THE HEALTH VISITOR IN CHILD ABUSE. JOINT STATEMENT. (British Association of Social Workers/Health Visitors' Association, 1982).

In this joint statement, it is recommended that a local authority social worker should usually be nominated as key worker in this context although in some cases this role may also be performed by a social worker from another setting, e.g. from the NSPCC. It was believed that the health visitor should not be nominated as a key worker since

health visitors did not have the appropriate resources or appropriate training to carry out some of
the tasks involved in acting as key worker. However, the statement did recommend

> that where the health visitor is the profes-
> sional most closely concerned with the case
> and is willing and in a position to undertake
> the responsibility for maintaining contact
> with the family, the role of key worker is to
> be divided into that of "prime worker" and
> "case co-ordinator".

The primeworker would be responsible for
'maintaining regular contact with the parents and
children appropriate to the health visiting needs
of the family, discussing with the family the outcome of case meetings (including registration) and
its implications', and 'keeping in regular contact
and discussing appropriate action with the case co-
ordinator' who should be a social worker of appropriately similar level. The case co-ordinator would
act as a central point of communication about the
case, make administrative arrangements for case
conferences and formally notify the family of decisions reached.

This statement therefore identified an appropriate role for the health visitor (namely prime
worker) but where it had been agreed that the role
of key worker was not divided into one of prime
worker and case co-ordinator, it should not be
undertaken by a member of the nursing profession
(including health visitors within this definition).

26. THINKING ABOUT HEALTH VISITING (Royal College
of Nursing, Society of Primary Health Care Nursing,
1983).

This document was produced in order to 'pro-
voke thinking and promote debate'. The following
factors or trends which underlie many of the problems and dilemmas in health visiting today are
identified, namely:

> the relationship between health visiting and
> maternal and child welfare;
> the relationship between health visiting and
> local authority services;
> the relationship between health visiting and
> primary medical care, in particular the eff-
> ects of its organisational system;

the administrative demarcation between health
and social services, and their increasing
specialisation and fragmentation of care;
the struggle of health visiting to "fit in" to
structural and policy changes which profoundly
affected it but were outside its control;
the problem of role definition in health visiting, particularly in relation to nursing and
social work;
the low priority accorded to prevention including the child health service within the
health services.

In a chapter entitled 'Health Visiting is
Nursing', the following problems were identified:

the shortcomings of the present system of
basic nursing training for the educational
preparation of health visitors;
the allocation of resources between health
visiting and other types of nursing services
within the nursing budget;
the control of health visiting services by all
managers who are not themselves experienced in
health visiting;
the difficulty experienced by health visitors,
who constitute a numerically small minority
group within nursing, in influencing nursing
policies;
the salary differentials which result from the
enhanced payments made for evening, night and
week-end work and hospital based clinical
teaching, which are not available for health
visitors;
the unequal relationship between nurses and
doctors especially in the acute hospital
setting;
the exclusive concentration on individual care
which may inhibit the health visitors' role in
community development.

Nevertheless the advisory group concluded, 'we believe that the advantages to health visiting of
greater integration within the profession of nursing greatly outweigh the disadvantages'.

Concerning 'Health Visiting in Primary Health
Care', the following issues were mentioned which
raised, the advisory group thought, a number of
questions to which health visitors should address
themselves:

How should the goals of primary health care and primary medical care be reconciled?
Is it possible to nurse (i.e. "foster the growth and development of") a community within the concept of attachment, which defines the team's clientele as a list of individuals?
How can primary prevention be promoted within a system dedicated to the cure or palliation of disease?
How can concepts such as "development of community resources" or "self reliance" be fostered within a model of care which depends on the concept of a professional/client relationship in which the professional may be seen by some to be dominant?
What alternative models of a primary health care team can be developed other than attachment, in order to meet the needs of areas where attachment is difficult to achieve?
How can the consumer of primary health care best participate in and contribute to, the primary health care services?

Concerning the heading 'Accountability and Standards of Practice', the following questions were identified which it was felt needed urgent consideration by health visitors themselves:

To whom is the health visitor accountable and for what?
What exactly is the health visitor's field of expertise within which she can be said to be competent and can therefore be held to be accountable?
How far is the health visitor an agent of social change or an agent of social control?
What constitutes an acceptable standard of health visiting service and health visiting practice?
How can health visitors individually and collectively ensure high standards of health visiting practice?

In the chapter entitled 'Approaches to Health Visiting Practice', among the issues raised were:

The importance of home visiting as a method of health visiting is taken for granted and is based to some extent on well established consumer expectations, but there appears to have been no systematic evaluation of

whether home visiting "works better" than alternative forms of contact. We subscribe to a
belief in the value of home visiting, but
since home visiting is a relatively expensive
form of service, it is important that it
should be subjected to more critical scrutiny.
As a starting point in this discussion we note
that in Finland health visiting is almost entirely clinic based, while in Denmark, health
visiting consists almost entirely of home visiting and clinics are used hardly at all. In
both countries, however, child health surveillance is more comprehensive than in the United
Kingdom. Can home visiting be justified as a
"method of health visiting" in its own right,
or only on the grounds that alternative settings are unavailable and unsuitable? What
are the consumers "demands" in regard to this
method of health visiting?
    ...One method of mobilising community
resources is the stimulation and development
of self-help groups and "lay" health workers.
.... As a method of health visiting should the
development of such groups and individuals be
encouraged?
    Another important issue in health visit-
ing practice is the degree to which specialisation is necessary or desirable. One of the
greatest strengths of health visiting is that
its specific skills are especially valuable
for tackling the widely differing health problems of people of all ages; paradoxically,
however, this may also be a major weakness
because the dissipation of these skills over
too wide a range reduces their effectiveness.
Although in practice the great majority of
health visiting work is undertaken with mothers and their children, health visitors see
themselves as generalists rather than specialists and see this as a major strength of
health visiting in an era of increasing specialisation and fragmentation in health care.
Should health visitors specialise more -
either in terms of work with particular groups
of people (e.g. the elderly) or in terms of
method (e.g. community development)? Can
health visitors acquire and maintain adequate
depth of knowledge in all fields? Should we
develop the concept of "consultancy" in health
visiting so that in addition to her work as a
generalist, a health visitor might develop

special expertise in one particular field which she then makes available on a consultancy basis to other health visitors? What are the implications of recommendations such as that of the Warnock Committee that the health visitor should be the key person in the care of the young handicapped child?

In the final chapter 'Health Visiting in Social Change', attention was drawn to the changes taking place in society, including changes in population structure, patterns of disease, the position of women, unemployment and technology (in particular information technology). The group also raised the issue of positive discrimination in a multi-racial, multi-cultural society, and concluded with the question:

Each of these issues - and the list is far from complete - demands careful consideration because each of them influences what health visiting is now, and what it could be. Taken together, however, such issues raise questions which are even more fundamental: how should health visiting respond to social change? - how far should health visitors support and maintain the status quo and how far should they actually promote change?

27. PROMOTING PREVENTION - A discussion document prepared by a working party of the Royal College of General Practitioners (the Royal College of General Practitioners, 1983).

The main aim of this document was to promote the concept of anticipatory care ('anticipatory care implies the union of prevention with care and cure - prevention including both the promotion of health and the prevention of disease'). The report clearly recognizes that anticipatory care is essentially a team activity involving community nurses amongst others. A number of its comments and suggestions do relate to community nurses and these are summarized or reproduced below.

Where resources have been made available to general practice, either through item-of-service payments or by the alignment of staff, general practitioners have shown themselves to be both capable of and willing to develop anticipatory care in their practices. Where res-

ources have not been available only enthus-
iasts have been able to find a way to pursue
their beliefs. The lesson should be obvious.
.... We suggest that every district health
authority develop a plan for primary care, including preventive services, and that this be
formulated by representatives of general practice, family practitioner committees, community health councils and those disciplines
making up the primary care team.

It was suggested that among the things that 'vocational trainees need to learn about health promotion, prevention of disease, self-care and the use
of medical services' are the following:

that he can describe the preventive role of
the health visitor and the district nurse and
that he can describe methods of strengthening
the primary care team.

The report endorses the recommendations generally of the Harding Report (1981) (see page 80 of
this book) and makes in particular the following
points:

Centrally we believe that the College should
foster closer links between health visitors,
midwives, nurses, social workers and representatives of ancillary staff, and that consideration be given to allowing them associate
membership. At the same time the faculties
should take the initiative in promoting a continuing dialogue with representatives from
other professions within the primary care
team.

The working party welcomed 'initiatives taken by
certain faculties in promoting educational courses
for practice managers' and felt 'that such initiatives could be expanded to promote interdisciplin-
ary training with midwives, health visitors and
district nurses.
In addition, on the specific subject of health
visitors and nurses, the following points were
made:

We are not clear about the aspirations
and the expectations of health visiting and
find the numerous references made to it by
those outside the profession confusing.

There is no doubt in our view that a much fuller and deeper examination of health visiting is needed and we applaud the health visitors in asking the Department of Health to appoint a team to undertake a comprehensive review - something that has not been done since 1958.

We are concerned that the training of health visitor students often takes place in isolation from the training of general practitioners, health education officers and community physicians, and suggest a need for a formal link between health visitor courses and academic departments of general practice or vocational training schemes.

We are not clear how district nursing sees its future evolution but feel that the new training for district nurses will equip them to make a broader contribution to prevention in the future.

Whilst we believe that the district nurse has a major contribution to make in the field of anticipatory care, especially in relation to the elderly and young chronic sick, we look to the nurses and health visitors to identify the respective contributions each profession can make and hope that in doing this they will consult with general practitioners and community physicians.

We believe that there should be much greater liaison between district nurse training programmes and vocational training schemes for general practice.

28. NURSE ALERT - A Report on the Effect of the Financial and Manpower Cuts in the NHS (Royal College of Nursing, 1984).

The Royal College of Nursing, a Trade Union and Professional Organisation with 232,000 members, launched its "nurse alert" campaign at the beginning of August 1983. It asked nurses to monitor the effects of the financial and manpower cuts imposed on the National Health Service...

...The College asked members in England through their local Centres to collate and corroborate information and then forward it to Headquarters. At the same time, the General Secretary wrote to regional and district nursing officers asking them to supply information about the scale of the cuts and how services might be affected

The report summarized the information received from these enquiries, certain of which relate specifically to community nursing facilities and is described below.

In the chapter headed 'New Demands for Health Care and Nursing manpower', it is pointed out that:

Although in 10 years the number of district nurses has risen by just over 3,000 - or by about 30 per cent - their official working week has also been reduced by six per cent and their holidays increased. In spite of this, district nurses have in 10 years, treated just over twice as many people and made half a million more home visits, the great majority of which were to people over 65 years [and it was thought that many of these were to the over 85s and likely to be time consuming]. Apart from the increase in the number of the aged, the district nurses are now treating twice the number of people physically handicapped or otherwise disabled under the age of 65 than they were doing 10 years ago. Again, such visits are time consuming and often physically hard. The Government's priority policy of community health services for the old and disabled is praiseworthy but is foundering on lack of manpower and lack of resource.

The report goes on to observe that the proportion of elderly in the population has steadily increased, and so have divorces with the result that a large number of children are being brought up by single parent families who tend to make greater demands on the community services.

Meanwhile there are fewer people in the median quartile to support and care for the old at home, particularly the old old, who will make great demands on the nursing services...
...The average family size is smaller, marriage or partnerships are earlier and there is increased mobility due to unemployment. There are therefore fewer relatives or long standing neighbours to help in time of trouble and it is common knowledge that health visit-

ors and district nurses are often turned to in
lieu of relatives...

It is also pointed out that there has been a
change in the morbidity patterns affecting the
demands for nursing care, for example a decline in
cases of infectious disease over the last thirty
years or so, matched by an increase in the numbers
of 'patients with multiple symptoms and disabilit-
ies which calls for a high degree of nursing skill
and knowledge and much evaluation.'
In the chapter headed 'What the Nurse Managers
Told Us' it was said that the point was often made
that the shortening of patients' stay in hospital

would place a greater strain on the already
stretched community services, but because of
manpower and revenue cuts no provision could
be made for an increase in the community
health staff or their resources. It was significant that in some places, the funding of
places for both district nurse training and
health visitor courses was being reduced and
newly qualified health visitors were unable to
find posts.

Reports from the Royal College of Nursing centres and from individual members also made similar
points in giving specific examples of problems.
The report concluded:

As far as community services are concerned,
there is a knock-on effect of delayed admissions and early discharge from hospital. It
is virtually impossible for the community services to turn away a patient.

29. TRAINING NEEDS OF PRACTICE NURSES. Report of
the Steering Group (Steering Group of the Royal
College of Nursing, Council for the Education and
Training of Health Visitors, Panel of Assessors for
District Nurse Training, Royal College of General
Practitioners and British Medical Association -
General Medical Services Committee, 1984).

The terms of reference of the steering group
were

to examine the training needs of practice
nurses and other nurses employed to work in
the treatment rooms of general practice or

> other health centre premises and to make
> recommendations.

The purpose of the report

> is to bring to the notice of the relevant
> authorities, the role and function of nurses
> working within general practice and health
> centre premises, to identify and specify the
> particular knowledge and skills with which
> they need to be equipped in order to function
> effectively, and to outline the structure and
> content of an appropriate educational pro-
> gramme.

From information available to the steering group,
there were now thought to be about 5,000 practice
nurses employed in England (in the context of the
total number of 11,000 general medical practices)
and that

> they were most numerous in the Midlands and
> Southern Counties and particularly in middle
> class areas such as Solihull, where more than
> half the practices employed a practice nurse.

The report observed that while 'the general practitioner employed nurse had the opportunity to negotiate her terms of service, role and function'
which allowed for flexibility that can meet the
requirements of individual medical practititioners
etc., the

> somewhat tenuous connection between these
> nurses and the National Health Service may
> limit their access to a range of educational
> opportunities which are taken for granted by
> the National Health Service employed nurses.

It was found that a number of courses had been
organized by various bodies for practice nurses,
financed by a variety of sources.

> Following representation by the General
> Medical Services Committee, the DHSS requested
> Area Health Authorities, as they then were, to
> allow practice nurses employed by general
> practitioners to attend without cost courses
> run by authorities for their own community
> nurses.

Significant DHSS and professional reports

...After further representations, the Statement of Fees and Allowances was amended so that the travelling and subsistence expenses of nurses attending such courses provided by health athorities could be reimbursed through the Family Practitioner Committee.

The steering group thought that:

there would seem to be a need for a centrally funded budget for all nursing education which would include the training of practice nurses.

The steering group recommended the following:

Nurses employed to work in general practice treatment rooms should receive specific training in accordance with the guidelines outlined in this report.
Courses for practice nurses should be planned in collaboration with local general practitioners and should, where possible be held in colleges of further and higher education alongside courses for district nurses and health visitors. Colleges should consider organising pilot courses for practice nurses and these might also be offered by postgraduate medical centres or health authorities.
Nurses currently employed as practice nurses should be given the opportunity to attend an appropriate course. Ultimately, courses for practice nurses should only be open to registered general nurses.

The steering group were of the opinion that:

in future the most appropriate initial qualification for entry to practice nursing would be at the level of registration. However nurses who are already employed should be offered training within the recommendations of this report.

This report includes guidelines on an outline curriculum and these we now reproduce, in parts in some detail, as it gives an insight into the kind of nursing that the steering group envisaged as being within the province of the practice nurse. The course content was to be based on three areas of study:

Professional role development
Procedures and techniques to be used in the treatment room/health centre
Management of the treatment room/health centre.

Areas to be studied under 'Professional Role Development' included the role and function of the practice nurse, the concept of the primary health care team and the roles of its members, counselling techniques and the health education of patients.

The report lists procedures and techniques required for the practice nurse working in the treatment room, including venepuncture, electro-cardiography screening techniques (which include taking blood pressures), first aid procedures and nursing care needed for minor ailments and infections.

Under the heading 'Practice Management and Administration' it was proposed that amongst other things this should include the structure and function of the Family Practitioner Committee; procedures for claiming fees and allowances; the use and function of age/sex and at risk registers; the use of computers in general practice; health and welfare of personnel; implications of the Health and Safety at Work Act, etc.; planning the layout of a treatment room in liaison with the architect.

The steering group made no recommendations as to the details of the length and pattern of the course, but thought it was unlikely that the content could be covered in less than ten full days. They thought that where possible such courses should be held alongside or 'interact with students of other disciplines with similar learning needs, i.e. district nurses, health visitors, practice managers, medical secretaries, general practitioners'.

The steering group recommended that:

validation of courses for practice nurses should be the responsibility of the new statutory nurse education bodies in order that a nationally recognised standard may be achieved.

30. FURTHER THINKING ABOUT HEALTH VISITING.
ACCOUNTABILITY IN HEALTH VISITING. A discussion
document (Health Visitors' Advisory Group of the
RCN Society of Primary Health Care Nursing, 1984).

This document took up the questions raised in
an earlier document produced by the same group,
entitled 'Thinking about Health Visiting' (see '
page 85), namely:

a. To whom is the health visitor accountable
and for what?
b. What exactly is the health visitor's
field of expertise within which she can be
said to be competent and can, therefore, be
held to be accountable?
c. How far is the health visitor an agent of
social change or an agent of social control?
d. What constitutes an acceptable standard
of health visiting service and health visiting
practice?
e. How can health visitors individually and
collectively ensure high standards of health
visiting practice?

Accountability was particularly an issue at
this time especially because of the publication of
the United Kingdom Central Council for Nursing,
Midwifery and Health Visiting's Code of Professional Conduct for Nurses, Midwives and Health visitors (1983) and because of

the appearance of a health visitor before the
UKCC's disciplinary committee, the first time
that a health visitor has been called to
account in respect of her position as a health
visitor.

A number of factors were mentioned as reasons
for the profession's increasing concern with accountability. These factors included:

the rising cost of health care and the consequent requirement to account for expenditure
and to justify services on the basis of value
for money and an increasingly better educated
public who demand a larger part in evaluating
the health care which they receive' and 'the
changed approach to nursing practice and nursing education exemplified by the use of the
nursing process and the increased range and

level of responsibility carried by nurses as a result of rapid expansion of the nursing role.

The advisory group described a framework for accountability - namely some concepts and the relationship between them - which was used in their analysis of the issue. Central to this notion was the concept of the <u>charge</u>: 'this represents the thing (decision, action) for which one is accountable.' 'The charge describes the content of each health visiting activity either actual or perceived.' It is crucially important that the charge be precisely defined for unless it 'is adequately specified it is not possible to talk about accountability for it'.

In order to be able to undertake the charge the health visitor requires the ability, responsibility and the authority to proceed.

<u>Ability</u> can mean not only, in the advisory group's opinion, knowledge, skills and values which are necessary to decide and act on specific issues but also the term must be taken to include resources - time, facilities and equipment and so on. 'Autonomy is an important facet of ability although it is also closely related to authority.'

<u>Responsibility</u> - 'this term is used for the giving or accepting of "the charge" and not to the charge itself...' 'In practice the source of responsibility in health visiting ... is the job description.'

<u>Authority</u> is defined as the 'rightful or legitimate power to fulfil a charge'. '...authority can be given but not taken.' There are three kinds of authority: authority of the situation - the right to do what needs to be done accorded to those present, for example, in an emergency, even though under other conditions such authority would not necessarily exist; the authority of expert knowledge which is to do with the 'formal recognition by society of professional expertise;' and the authority of position or structural authority 'is represented in nursing by a system of "line management"'. It was contended that the first of these three types of authority is not usually accorded to health visitors.

Finally, <u>accountability</u> is defined simply as 'being answerable, having to answer for one's decisions or actions'. The accountability question is then redefined as follows:

Significant DHSS and professional reports

To whom is the health visitor accountable and
for what and why?
How can this accountability be demonstrated or
put into practice?

The advisory group comments that

the means of demonstrating that a job has been
done in health visiting (that is, that the
charge has been fulfilled) is that it has been
documented. It is for this reason that health
visiting records are so important.

The advisory group then relates these concepts of
charge, ability, responsibility, authority and
accountability, to a variety of health visiting
activities, under the following headings:

Providing a service to a population
The advisory group stated that the charge for
the individual health visitor needs to be more
clearly specified than is now usual, and the population to be given a service by the health visitor
must be clearly defined. They stressed the importance of the health visitor participating in policy
decisions about 'the amount and type of services to
be provided'. At managerial level, the group noted
that quantitative accounting for the work done by
health visitors was relatively easy, the difficulty
lay in accounting for the quality of the service.
They reported that

At present the indicator most used by health
authorities and health service managers is
negative criticism, namely the number of complaints received from users of the services.

Accountability in health visiting practice
The group stated that the health visitor was
accountable firstly to the client, whether 'individual, family or group'. In considering home visiting by the health visitor, they thought that
'specifying the charge could also be a collab-
orative activity', in which the health visitor
could make her goals and the service she is offering more explicit to the client. The group approved of the more widespread use of 'the nursing
process' in health visiting and suggested that
records should be shared with clients.
The importance of keeping records was stressed, although the present systems were seen as in-

adequate and the group wanted to see the 'speedy implementation of the recommendations of the Körner Committee'. They also 'believed that systems of auditing and peer review ... could be developed in health visiting'.

Turning their attention to the work of the health visitor in the clinic, the group noted that much of this work had been taken over by staff other than health visitors. This in turn raised the problem of accountability (in contrast to the situation where the health visitor makes a home visit) if for instance an abnormality in a baby is not detected in the clinic and the baby was not seen by the health visitor.

Teamwork: shared accountability

The group was concerned with accountability when the health visitor is a member of a team, and in particular when she is a member of the primary health care team. The health visitor is 'exclusively occupied in preventive health care' and her 'charge' needs to be recognized by all the team. Where one member of the team is in frequent contact with a family, the advisory group suggest that this member should become the 'key worker' for the family, co-ordinating care with other members, for instance in the management of minor illness in children.

The work of the health visitor in child health surveillance and with the elderly was considered by the group, as it demonstrated the complexity of accountability when both health visitors and other professional workers are involved. The group felt that the health visitor should have the greater part of the responsibility and accountability for child health surveillance, and that in this sphere health visitors could demonstrate their accountability by 'measures such as audit and peer group review'. It was emphasized that the health visitor was not simply concerned with detecting abnormalities by screening children, but with reviewing a child's 'material, social and intellectual environment'.

The group felt that the work of health visitors with the elderly was limited, not just by the preference of many health visitors for work with children and their less developed 'knowledge base' about the elderly, but also because of limited resources and inadequate administrative systems, for instance the health visitor could not 'mobilize the support services, such as a home help, for which authority is vested in the social services department'.

Accountability to clients: the role of the patient advocate

The advisory committee believed that the role of patient advocate was central to that of the health visitor even though it was not always recognized by some health visitors and some employing authorities.

Client advocacy has two goals:

> The first is to help clients gain greater independence. The community health nurse shows clients what services are available, which they are entitled to, and how to obtain them until they can discover this information for themselves. A second goal is to help make the system more responsive and relevant to the needs of clients. By calling attention to inadequate or unjust care, the community health nurse can influence change.

The group

> recognised that this charge is one of the most difficult for the health visitor to fulfil because it is fraught with conflict arising from the health visitor's multiple accountabilities.

Finally in the conclusions of this document, it is mentioned that:

> Some strategies have been suggested which health visitors might explore as a means of achieving accountability in practice, in particular improved documentation, the use of the nursing process, audit, and peer group review.

31. NEIGHBOURHOOD NURSING - A FOCUS FOR CARE (DHSS, 1986).

The government appointed the Community Nursing Review Team chaired by Mrs Julia Cumberlege in June 1985 with the following terms of reference:

> To study the nursing services provided outside hospital by Health Authorities, and to report to the Secretary of State on how resources can

be used more effectively, so as to improve the services available to client groups. The input from nurses employed by general practitioners will be taken into account.

The team summarized its recommendations as follows:

1. Each district health authority should identify within its boundaries neighbourhoods for the purposes of planning, organising and providing nursing and related primary care services.
2. A neighbourhood nursing service (NNS) should be established in each neighbourhood.
3. Each neighbourhood nursing service should be headed by a manager chosen for her management skills and leadership qualities, and she should be based in the neighbourhood.
4. Community midwives, community psychiatric nurses and community mental handicap nurses should ensure, through their respective managers and the neighbourhood nursing manager, that their specialist contributions are fully co-ordinated with the work of the neighbourhood nursing service.
5. All other specialist nurses who work outside hospital should be based in the community and managed as part of the neighbourhood nursing service. Each specialist nurse should be assigned to one or more neighbourhood services and have the commitment of her time to each service specified.
6. The principle should be adopted of introducing the nurse practitioner into primary health care.
7. The DHSS should agree a limited list of items and simple agents which may be prescribed by nurses as part of a nursing care programme, and issue guidelines to enable nurses to control drug dosage in well-defined circumstances.
8. To establish and be recognised as a primary health care team, each general medical practice and the community nurses associated with it should come to an understanding of the team's objectives and individuals' roles within it.

That understanding should be incorporated into a written agreement signed jointly by the practice partners and by the manager of the neighbourhood nursing service on behalf of the relevant health authority.

The agreement should name the doctors and community nurses who together form the primary care team and should guarantee the right of the team members to be consulted on any changes proposed in its composition.

The making of such an agreement should be a qualifying condition for any incentive payments which may be introduced to improve quality in general practice (as suggested in the recent policy statement of the Royal College of General Practitioners).

9. The Government should invite the Health Advisory Service, with its established reputation, credibility and acceptance by the professions, to take on responsibility for identifying and promoting good practice in primary health care.

10. Subsidies to general practitioners enabling them to employ staff to perform nursing duties should be phased out.

11. Within two years, the United Kingdom Central Council for Nursing, Midwifery and Health Visiting and the English National Board should introduce a common training course for all first-level nurses wishing to work outside hospital in what are now the fields of health visiting, district nursing and school nursing.

12. The provision of nursing services in the community should remain the responsibility of district health authorities. We would urge, however, that in due course the Government should give consideration to amalgamating family practitioner committees and district health authorities and so bring all primary health care services under the control of one body.

13. A short but thorough manpower planning exercise on a practical (as distinct from purely academic) basis should be undertaken to ensure that the training and supply of community nurses, is, and remains at, the appropriate level. The

study should be supported by the NHS
Management Board as an essential task in
reviewing the adequacy and consistency of
Regional Plans.

14. Health care associations should be
formed, each covering one or more neighbourhoods.

In the foreword, the following points were
made:

We started from the premise that people
pay an average of £290 each year for their
National Health Service and so are entitled to
receive a service they want as well as need
.... Any successful service industry must regularly undertake market research to decide how
it should develop...

...We are not calling for more resources,
but a switch of resources within the NHS and
better use of existing funds to enable people
to have a realistic choice of being cared for
at home rather than in a hospital or other
institution...

However the danger is that if more people
are treated at home the resources needed to
keep them properly cared for may not be swit-
ched from hospital services to the community.
Voices of health staff and vulnerable people
scattered throughout the community may not be
strong enough to prevail over those who demand
unlimited resources for high technology medicine. The economy of looking after people at
home becomes more apparent once a whole hospital is closed but we see no reason why
health authorities should not identify community services as a first call on their
funds.

The cornerstone of our report, as its
title indicates, is a recommendation that in
each District neighbourhood nursing services
should be established. Health visitors, district nurses and school nurses, with their
support staff would thus provide a strong,
closely integrated, locally managed service
near to the consumer. We suggest that such
neighbourhoods should comprise between 10,000
and 25,000 people.

We found that nurses are at their most
effective when they and general practitioners
work together in an active primary health care

team. This is the best means of delivering comprehensive care to the consumer, but in many places the primary health care team is more a concept than a reality. We believe it has a greater chance of being a reality if doctors and nurses are encouraged to enter into formal agreements to establish and maintain care teams. The basis of such agreements between the neighbourhood nursing service and the doctors' practices would be that the aims and objectives, methods of working and monitoring of the total service would be negotiated and agreed by both parties. We believe that teams developed in this way would make full use of the skills of each member, adopt efficient working practices and, with regular review of performance, give people better health care. We outline in our report the potential advantages of these agreements not only to nurses but also to general practitioners and how the fuller use of nurses' skills can make both the doctor's and the nurse's job more satisfying. Where general practitioners eschew the team concept the neighbourhood nursing service would make provision for nursing care.

We gave a great deal of thought to the position of practice nurses. They are employed by general practitioners to carry out many tasks which the doctors feel community nurses are not always able to do because their priorities and accountability lie elsewhere. Employing a practice nurse entitles a general practitioner to claim a 70 per cent subsidy. If all general practitioners in England took advantage of their full entitlement the number of practice nurses could escalate by another 20,000 at a cost of more than £100 million a year. This would lead increasingly to the growth of a separate and fragmented nursing workforce in the community. Moreover, many community nurses are justifiably annoyed when asked to do work for which general practitioners receive payment through "item of service" arrangements. This means the NHS is paying nearly twice-over for a single task. For both these reasons we recommend that the subsidy should be phased out.

We would like to see the subsidy redirected into strengthening the community nursing service, not least through the introduction into primary health care of the nurse practitioner. She would work alongside doctors, would be responsible to them for agreed medical protocols, and be available for direct consultation by patients.

We also recommend that community nurses should be able to prescribe a limited range of items and simple agents and to control drug dosage in certain well-defined circumstances. This may require some legislation but in general we have tried to avoid anything that would involve changes in the law.

We came firmly to the opinion that in future nurses should undergo a common training for work in the community. We recognise the need for specialist nurses, but we were unhappy (as many nurses are) about health visitors, district nurses and school nurses being hemmed inside their own particular professional disciplines. The divisions these create neither serves the interests of the public nor gives community nurses the freedom and scope to use their full range of skills.

The Review Team recommends that for the time being community nurses should be managed by district health authorities. We rejected suggestions that family practitioner committees should be reorganised to do the job and that general practitioners should employ and manage nurses. In the long term we would prefer to see the roles and responsibilities of family practitioner committees and district health authorities combined to give a more cost-effective and coherent service.

At the centre of the recommendations are several proposals relating to the organization of community nursing and its relationships with other parts of the health service, but in particular there is the proposal that a team of community nurses serve a geographical area and that the team define its professional links, and more particularly its primary health care team activities, with local general practitioners, via a formal agreement. This was in preference to attachment arrangements of a kind whereby a community nurse's 'population of clients' were defined as being the patients on the list of one or more general practitioners - except where the zoning of general practitioners led to matching practice areas and neighbourhoods (or sub-neighbourhoods). It was proposed that the neighbourhood nursing team should be managed by line 'neighbourhood nursing managers' and a number of special activities suggested which such managers might undertake as part of their duties in managing nursing in a neighbourhood. In particular,

The neighbourhood nursing manager should:
be fully trained in management skills;
identify gaps in community health care provision and propose how they should be closed;
determine and know how to use the management information required to identify local needs and to evaluate the effectiveness of nursing services in meeting them;
have some clinical nursing responsibilities which will help to ensure that her professional skills are maintained and respected by her staff;
ensure that individual community nurses are achieving agreed objectives in their day-to-day work;
advise on professional development and further training;
determine and co-ordinate ways of working with specialist care teams, social services, local voluntary organisations and self-help groups;
deal with suggestions and complaints from consumers.

The neigbourhood nursing manager, it was recommended, should be locally and accessibly based and would meet frequently with local general practitioners and others concerned with community nurses in the provision of primary health care.

The proposal that reimbursement of part of the cost to the general practitioner of employing practice nurses should be phased out represents a further suggestion for rationalizing the provision of nursing services in the community. The report expresses the belief that within neighbourhood nursing teams:

...the professional demarcation lines of responsibility which have existed for so long would fade at last, and the staff would exploit much more flexibly and fully those skills they have which at present go unused.

This could mean many health visitors rediscovering and using some of the practical skills they acquired in their nurse training; it could mean school nurses using their counselling and health education skills outside schools with people other than school children; it could mean district nurses supervising preventive screening programmes for "well adults" or elderly people.

The report also gives attention to the relationship of core members of the neighbourhood nursing team, namely district nurses, health visitors and school nurses (plus their supporting staff) with specialist nurses working in the community. It proposes that except where (as in the case of community midwifery and psychiatric nursing) there are good reasons for integrating hospital and community care within those particular disciplines, specialist nurses serving the community should be based in and managed as part of community services.

The review team proposed that neighbourhood nursing and other community nursing services should be managed within the district health authority (rather than, for example, their being transferred to family practitioner committees) though they did propose the amalgamation of the family practitioner committees and district health authorities in the longer term.

One modification in the roles of community nurses, namely a suggestion of greater flexibility, has already been noted. Two further recommendations of significance were made. The first of these was that the nurse practitioner should be introduced into primary health care.

We believe that community nurses who have, or acquire, the necessary skills in health promotion and the diagnosis and treatment of disease among people of all ages should have the opportunity to practise those skills in the setting of a clinic in the neighbourhood.

We are not proposing they should become mini-doctors. We are suggesting that patients who visit their general practitioners with conditions which are self-limiting, or want to discuss another aspect of their health care, should have a choice of whom to see. Research has shown that nurses can be as effective as doctors - and as acceptable to patients - in securing compliance with therapy for chronic disease, making initial assessments of patients, diagnosing and treating certain minor acute illnesses and behavioural disorders, and rehabilitating elderly people after surgery.

The second and related recommendation was in connection with the power to prescribe:

> We found district nurses waste time in requesting prescriptions from general practitioners for such things as dressings, ointments and medical sprays - those for leg ulcers, for example.
>
> In addition, many nurses have become very skilled in managing pain relief programmes for terminally ill patients. We believe therefore that community nurses who work with terminally ill patients should be permitted to use their professional judgement on matters such as the timing and dosage of drugs prescribed for pain relief... This may require nurses carrying their own supply of drugs as midwives do now.

The other recommendations of the report included those concerned with education for a new pattern of nursing in the community, means of assuring and maintaining quality, and of ensuring an adequate supply of human resources necessary to staff the service.

The overall impact of the recommendations if implemented, particularly those based on the neighbourhood nursing team, would be in a sense to establish nursing as a distinct and perhaps most basic unit of health provision within the community - as the only group with responsibility for caring for everyone in a relatively specific small geographical area in contrast with the general practitioners providing services to specific individuals.

The second half of the report consisted of a detailed action programme for establishing neighbourhood nursing services and the provision of services for the various categories of patients within the context of such teams.

32. PRIMARY HEALTH CARE: AN AGENDA FOR DISCUSSION. (DHSS et al. 1986).

This discussion paper was published at the same time as the Cumberlege Report (Neighbourhood Nursing - A Focus for Care, see page 101) and was primarily concerned with family practitioner services. It did however relate specifically to some

of the recommendations in the report of the community nursing review team (the Cumberlege Report).
    In chapter ten: 'Community Nursing Services',
the recommendations of the Cumberlege Report are
summarized and generally speaking it was indicated
that 'the government intends that there be discussion and comment on that report as part of the
primary care debate in England'. However, in the
case of three specific issues, an indication was
given of the government's thinking as follows.
Firstly it was stated regarding GP employed nurses
that 'the government does not intend to end the
present arrangement of part direct and part in-
direct reimbursement of the cost'. Secondly, as
regards the recommendation that consideration be
given to amalgamating family practitioner committees and district health authorities, it was stated
that 'it was too soon to contemplate changes, which
would in any case, need to be based on a close
analysis of the likely benefits'. The third matter
was that of the possibility of a salaried family
doctor service. Concerning this it was stated that
'the government believes that the independent contractor status of family doctors has brought benefits and should continue.'
    It was stated that five main themes identified
from the Cumberlege Report's recommendations should
be discussed, namely:

        neighbourhood nursing services;
        making better use of nursing skills;
        improving the effectiveness of the primary
        health care team;
        changes in nurse training;
        increasing public involvement in the way
        services are run.

    Turning to the recommendations on the general
practitioner services, no radical changes were envisaged though changes in detail in the way general
practitioners were remunerated to provide incen-
tives to good practice were suggested. Other recommendations which have some bearing on community
nursing were that the government wished to increase
the numbers of family doctors involved in community
child health care and wished to encourage developments in the prevention of ill-health and the promotion of good health.
    Concerning the role of pharmacists,

the government believes there is scope for
making better use of pharmacy skills in advising patients and providing other services both
for patients and doctors' and 'will examine
carefully and positively what additional contribution pharmacies might make to NHS primary
care.

The discussion paper floated the idea of
'health care shops':

The development of integrated schemes offering
the full range of primary health care services
is currently inhibited by regulations prevent-
ing anyone other than a dentist or doctor from
running a dental business for profit. There
are no similar rules in relation to other
primary care professions and provided there
are safeguards for professional standards, its
removal may open the way to new schemes under
which more than one service is provided under
the same roof - such as health care "shops".

Chapter Four

DEVELOPMENTS IN THE LAST DECADE AND SOME IDEAS FOR THE FUTURE

INTRODUCTION

In this chapter we review schemes and studies in community nursing which have been described in the literature since 1974, and we have supplemented these descriptions with information obtained from our postal survey of chief nursing officers in England. (See Chapter One for details of how we obtained information from all these sources.) Many schemes and studies reflect ideas put forward or tried out prior to 1974, and so in that sense are not completely 'new'; however, they do give some idea of the development and popularity of these ideas since 1974.

We have been primarily concerned with developments in community nursing in England, but in the literature referred to we have included items from the United Kingdom, and particularly from Scotland. We have aimed to cover the range and variety of schemes and studies we found, not necessarily including every single example of a particular type of development.

At the end of the chapter we look at ideas for future developments in community nursing which we obtained from the literature, from the survey of chief nursing officers, and from discussion with professionals in this field.

The chapter is divided into six main parts, namely:

Health visiting
District nursing
Practice nurses
Extending the role of the nurse
General reviews of schemes and studies
Ideas for future developments

Some of these six parts are further divided into sections and sub-sections. In the first five parts describing schemes and studies, we consider first the literature on the subject and then, for each part (or section or sub-section if the part is so divided) we briefly sum up what was reported from the survey of chief nursing officers on the same subject. (The survey is referred to as the 'CNO survey' for the sake of brevity.) One hundred and forty-three CNOs of health authorities in England (74% of those approached) responded to the survey. Their replies give information on developments in their authorities as at late 1982 and early 1983. It may be that, not only have there been new developments since then in these health districts, but also that some schemes may have been discontinued, as many schemes were subject to assessment or dependent on sufficient funds being allocated to them.

HEALTH VISITING

Organizational aspects of health visiting
The main change in the organization of health visiting (and indeed in district nursing) which has occurred in recent years is the move to attachment schemes. Attachment to general practices, which was the subject of several studies before 1974, has become the norm, although it is being questioned.

A study carried out by Dawtrey (1976) compared the work of attached and unattached health visitors working from two health centres in inner London. She found that although the breadth of cases presented to the health visitor was influenced by whether she was attached or unattached, a number of factors including the organizational structure of the building she worked from and its design affected her methods of helping. Dawtrey states that:

Attachment can provide opportunities for the delivery of a comprehensive, effective primary health care system but the important role of the unattached health visitor must not be excluded. Many sections of urban society do not settle in one community for any length of time and certainly do not register with a general practitioner, without the work of the unattached health visitor, this group would fall through the primary health care net.

Poulton (1977) undertook an extensive study of health visitors and district nurses in the Wandsworth and East Merton Teaching District. She distinguished between 'attachment' ('nurses practising and working with general practitioners from health centres or group practices') and 'alignment' ('nurses working with a number of general practitioners in various practices but based at centres'). She found that 'the aligned health visitor spends more time on client visits including routine visits' while the 'attached health visitor spends more time in consultation with the general practitioner'. Under both arrangements she found that the health visitor spent about half her working time on administrative work (mainly 'writing reports, preparing forms and statistics and making/receiving telephone calls'). She found that even amongst attached health visitors professional contact with general practitioners was low and felt that communications between district nurses and health visitors could be strengthened. She recommended that attached schemes should be developed on the basis of 'confined attachment areas' and where this is not possible 'geographical organisation of workload may be a solution'. In either event she advocated district nurses and health visitors should be allocated to a conterminous geographical area.

Another study (Walsworth-Bell, 1979) compared the work of health visitors in two adjacent health districts. In one district, health visitors were all attached, in the other, most worked on a geographical basis. The work of the two groups was remarkably similar but some differences emerged. In the geographical district, the health visitors were more likely to make contact with patients 'in the street or in houses which were not the home of the primary patient', they did more follow-up visits, in particular they did more follow-ups to households without a registered general practitioner. It was planned to experiment with a mixed scheme, with attached health visitors having territorial responsibilities.

Gilmore et al.(1974) carried out a major study of health visitors and district nurses in primary health care teams looking at a number of factors relating to the development of teamwork. One of the most interesting ideas explored in practice was that of the 'nursing co-ordinator' of the team. This was one of the health visitors or district nurses in the team whose function was to facilitate the smooth working of the team - in particular it

was not a line management role. In one of the
three teams studied intensively, the nurse co-
ordinator was also Chairman of the Practice Committee, comprising the general practitioners as
well.

One part of the country which had health visitor shortages was Thanet, Kent, where a 'flexibank' of health visitors and SRN assistants was set
up (Bolton, 1981). The systems enabled a crisis
service to be maintained, with priority for babies
and young children. It is concluded that although
the flexibank enabled the population to have basic
health visitor services, it was only for use in a
crisis, and was no substitute for routine visiting
and record keeping, and responsibility for a known
caseload.

Clode (1978) referred to an experiment in
Trafford Area Health Authority where health visitors were integrated into a 'preventive' division
rather than the usual community division, emphasizing their preventive role as opposed to the curative function of other community services. Finance
for the 'preventive' division, which also includes
health education, family planning, school and child
health services, was achieved by transferring money
from the hospitals, as assessed by their bed occup-
ancy. As a result of this, it was reported that the
health visitor to population ratio had improved,
with more visits being made, reduced caseloads and
no problems filling vacancies. This arrangement
was unusual in that health visitors came under a
different division to the community nursing services.

Two studies have been concerned with the
effect of routine clerical work on the use of the
health visitor's time. A survey in North Stafford-
shire Health Authority was made (Watts, 1985) of 19
health visitors who completed time sheets and questionnaires. The survey showed that 'about one-
fifth of time was taken up by routine clerical
work, despite the fact that almost all health visitors had some clerical help available', and this
routine work could be undertaken by less highly
trained persons.

A pilot scheme was introduced in Bexley Health
Authority 'to test the hypothesis that relieving
health visitors of basic clerical duties will improve the quality of client care and provide financial savings' (O'Connor and Willis, 1985). It
had been 'estimated that effective clerical support
would reduce the office time of each health visitor

by 17 per cent', and ten whole time equivalent
health visitors and four clerical staff took part
in the scheme. Targets for performance were agreed
with the health visitors concerned, such as increased visiting to priority groups, as well as a
decrease in office time of at least 17 per cent.
With the increased clerical support, the health
visitors achieved almost all the targets, and saved
even more office time than expected. As a result,
the scheme has been implemented throughout the
health authority.

Nine health authorities in the CNO survey referred to their arrangements - attachment or other
systems - for health visiting staff. Two authorities (Barnsley and Hillingdon) had changed back to
a geographical system. Hillingdon reported that
the general practitioners were not happy with this
arrangement but that

> the health visitors feel they are functioning
> more effectively geographically and have no
> wish to return to attachment until the general
> practitioners have a greater understanding of
> the role of the health visitor.

In Coventry health visitors were both 'aligned' to
practices and in addition had a geographical
'patch'.

A London authority (West Lambeth) reported
that they had negotiated with a neighbouring authority (Camberwell) that health visitors would cover
all GP practice patients, whichever authority the
patients lived in.

In some Leicestershire towns, health visitors
were based together with other community nurses, in
cottage hospitals.

Health visitors providing services out of normal
hours

Some studies have described and/or evaluated
health visitor services outside normal hours, usually for parents with young children.

A 'crying baby' advisory service for 'out-of-
hours' times was introduced at Huddersfield in 1977
experimentally and kept on after evaluation. Some
other places have followed suit. At Richmond (London) a scheme for telephone advice at weekends
about crying babies was started and has been kept
on as an 'essential' service (Beech, 1981). Another
crying baby advice service was tried out at Ply-
mouth (Bogie, 1981) but although the health visit-

ors were convinced of its value, general practitioners and midwives were not and the future of the
whole scheme was in the balance. Subsequently although thought to be a very useful scheme, it was
eventually abandoned, for like many other districts
it was not considered a priority in terms of funding. In Preston a 24-hour service for telephone advice by health visitors on child health problems
generally, was set up as a pilot scheme (Metcalf,
et al. 1981). This was judged as a success and
kept on as part of the normal health visitor service.

The aims of such schemes are not only preventive (e.g. to prevent possible 'battering') but
also cost-saving since it is reported that many
patients would have called out a general practitioner, if the advice service from health visitors
had not been available. This latter aim is difficult to prove as it depends on what the client said
they would do otherwise, and of course sometimes
the general practitioner had to be called in anyway. However, there seemed to be widespread approval of these schemes by the health visitors and
families concerned.

In Peterborough, some of the health visitors
operate a telephone rota system in order to provide
seven day cover (Rawdon Smith, 1984). A health
visitor is on telephone duty at a health centre for
an hour in the mornings at weekends and bank holidays to take calls which she then follows up by
visits if necessary. Clients themselves, other
health visitors, the paediatric and maternity departments of the hospital, social services, and nursing management have all made referrals via this
system. Most of these referrals concern young babies, and it is felt that the workload generated at
weekends (244 referrals resulting in 215 visits in
the first year) shows the need for such a scheme.
The scheme is not expensive as for each of the half
days worked at weekends, a weekday is taken off in
lieu by the health visitor concerned.

Another variation on out-of-hours work is provided by Enfield health visitors (Haylock, 1981 and
Anon., 1982). They are not only on call out-of-
hours for emergencies but also do some routine work
in the evenings, which is more convenient for some
families, e.g. if both parents are out during the
day. The health visitors operating the scheme are
specifically recruited for out-of-hours work and
are provided with GPO radiopaging devices so they
can be 'bleeped' wherever they may be in the dis-

trict. A child health clinic was tried on one Saturday morning for each month, but had to be discontinued owing to lack of clinical medical officer time.

Finally another variation on this theme - Sheffield local radio services (both BBC and commercial) have put on 'phone-in' programmes for parents to put questions to health care professionals about child health problems (Anon., 1979).

Five health authorities responding to the CNO survey mentioned their schemes for health visitors providing services out-of-hours. Of these, three (in Huddersfield, Peterborough and Preston) were the schemes already referred to in the literature review above. In addition an 'on-call system' for mothers with child rearing problems operates in North West Durham, and in Medway health visitors are on call for mothers and would make visits in the evening.

Health visitors and the elderly

One continuing pre-occupation which is apparent from the literature is the role of the health visitor in relation to the elderly. The survey for the OPCS by Dunnell and Dobbs (1982) found only 9% of the health visitors' time was spent with those of 65 or over, but that health visitor assistants spent 57% of their time with the same age group. In this section we look first at schemes for the screening and surveillance of the elderly which involve health visitors and then at liaison and 'intervention' schemes.

a)   Health visitors and the screening and surveillance of the elderly. A number of studies have been done in which the health visitor was involved in screening for problems among elderly patients. This is not a new idea - there are reports on this from pre-1974 - but it is still a subject for study, and all the more relevant now with increasing numbers of elderly in the population.

In one study in a general practice in Scotland, a health visitor, using a specially devised questionnaire, visited a randomly selected sample of those aged 70 and over and the information she obtained was compared to an assessment of the same patients by a geriatrician and an assessment by the general practitioner using his knowledge of the patient (Powell and Crombie, 1974). There was mostly a good correlation between the health visitor's assessments of the physical and mental state of the patients compared to that of the doctors. The authors felt that a community nurse could use such a questionnaire effectively for screening the elderly.

Another Scottish study (Gardiner, 1975) also used a questionnaire administered by health visitors, to assess medical and social needs of patients in a group practice who were aged 75 and over. In addition some basic clinical tests were made. The study found that 82% of the 237 elderly persons visited had 'some significant pathology' and calculated that to maintain the surveillance and meet the needs arising, there would have to be expansion in 'medical, nursing, dental, laboratory and social work' resources.

Health visitors and district nurses undertook a survey of the over-80 age group registered with an urban practice in Yorkshire (Heath and Fitton, 1975). The staff did this in addition to normal duties, using an interview to obtain information about the health, social state and environment of the patient. There was no 'urgent concealed medical need' found but the survey did find some health and social needs and felt that surveillance of the age group was essential.

Barber and Wallis (1976) describe a system introduced into a health centre in Glasgow where the health visitor in the practice made an assessment of the elderly (65 plus) patients already in contact with the general practitioner or health visitor. The carrying out of assessments did not need extra staff, although they did generate extra workload as a result of problems identified. Health visitors felt that visits based on these assessments were more useful than previous visits had been.

Later on the same team tested a postal questionnaire to screen a sample of the elderly (70 and over), not just those already with the general practitioner and health visitor. They concluded that the questionnaire was acceptable to patients, it identified patients who could benefit from further assessment by the health visitor, and reduced the workload that would be needed for routine assessment by visiting (Barber, Wallis and McKeating, 1980). They developed the questionnaire to use it on all patients of 65 or over in a practice which had used no screening procedures at all (Barber and Wallis, 1982). Two part-time research health visitors carried out the screening and assessment, and the workload of the primary care team was monitored

before, during and after the period of 'intervention' by screening and assessment. It was found
that workload with the elderly for doctors, nurses
and health visitors rose substantially during the
'intervention' phase. After this phase the general
practitioner workload dropped considerably, but although the district nurse and health visitor workload with the elderly decreased, it was still
higher than before 'intervention'. As a result of
the assessments made, 78% of elderly patients were
found to have 'unrecognized or unreported problems
or symptoms'. It was concluded that the extra work
which would be needed for an attached health visit-
or to routinely undertake screening and assessment
for patients of 70 and 75 years and over was not
excessive and time well spent.

The geriatric assessment form developed by
Barber and his colleagues in the studies described
above, was also used in another study conducted in
Cumbernauld New Town in Scotland (Smith, Robertson
and Bishop, 1984). The health visitor or her aide
set out to visit all patients in the practice of 65
or over, and ultimately interviewed 70% of this age
group in their homes. The survey found few serious
medical problems but did find 'a considerable number of social and environmental problems', which
were mostly successfully helped.

A survey of all the elderly registered with a
practice was done in Glasgow (Currie et al. 1974)
by a health visitor and a nurse, for patients aged
70-72. They visited the patients at home and the
general practitioner subsequently examined them.
It was concluded that an extra health visitor or
nurse is needed by a practice of three or four
general practitioners to do this type of work, and
in fact little serious morbidity was uncovered.

A scheme in Reading (Curnow et al. 1975) used
specially appointed health visitors to identify
those over 65 who had health or social needs, who
would benefit from help. Unfortunately not all
needs could be met with the resources available,
and it was not a satisfying full-time occupation
for the health visitors. Some improvements in
local services were made as a result. This scheme
does raise a basic problem about any survey for
need, namely of caring agencies being able to cope
with the demands that arise as a result. (The same
study is described from the point of view of the
interviewing health visitor by Livingston, 1974.)

One practice has undertaken a two month pilot
scheme for visiting the 70-and-over age group in

which a health visitor makes a first assessment
visit and an SEN does follow-up visits. The SEN
does some basic clinical tests but subsequently is
also involved with arranging social support for
those in need (Neil, 1982). The scheme is described as a success and is being continued.

Similarly in a practice in Suffolk, a health
visitor assistant (SRN) has carried out assessment
visits to the 75-year-old and over patients in the
practice, supervized by the health visitor (Black,
1984). Many patients were reported to have been
given help for minor medical and social problems as
a result, and were encouraged to make further self-
referrals if necessary. The assessment visits were
also intended to provide some health education material, but patients were not receptive to this. The
scheme is being continued, extending the age range
to 70, and with the intention of doing repeat assessments in due course.

A geriatric liaison health visitor has described a survey of patients aged 80 or more registered with one general practitioner which she
undertook (Joyce, 1985). She visited them at home,
assessing their social situation, environmental
hazards, and health. Apart from asking questions,
the health visitor also took blood pressures and
tested urine. Half of those surveyed (63 patients)
needed some action on their behalf, and most needs
could be met. It was hoped that the same type of
survey could be done by the geriatric liaison
health visitor for other practices, and to repeat
it in two or three years time.

A study was made in the Lisburn Unit of Management in Northern Ireland to find out 'whether or
not the services provided for the elderly population were fully meeting their needs' (Wightman,
1985). Two health visitors were selected to visit
patients aged 65 or more, initially in one general
practice as a pilot study. The two health visitors, together with two staff nurses, then moved to
other practices (with the agreement of the general
practitioners) 'to identify for the practice health
visitor, those elderly clients most at risk'. Needs
identified and referrals were dealt with by the
team of health visitors and staff nurses, which was
known as the 'health maintenance team'. A micro-
computer was used in the survey, reducing clerical
time. The initial survey identified unmet needs in
over 36% of the patients, and a system of review
for patients over 65 at two or three yearly intervals has been instituted, using visits, clinical

assessments and postal questionnaires. Research is showing 'a decreasing number of needs on the second, third and subsequent reviews of practices'.

However, not all reported surveys of the elderly agree that the results of screening are worthwhile. Freedman et al. (1978) carried out a comprehensive screening of all patients over 65 in their Newcastle-upon-Tyne practice. It was feared that because of the decline in home visiting by the general practitioner, health and social problems might be missed. They concluded that the screening procedure revealed 'little treatable but previously undiagnosed illness' and that the lack of visits to the elderly by the general practitioner was offset by more visiting from district nurses and health visitors.

Seven health authorities responding to the CNO survey reported having screening or assessment schemes for the elderly which involved health visitors; in one of these (in Bloomsbury) patients aged 55 and over who had not seen a general practitioner for a year were approached by the health visitor or geriatric visitor.

b) Health visitors and the elderly - liaison and 'intervention' schemes. Health visitor skills have also been used apart from screening to give special attention to the needs of the elderly. In one London borough, a health visitor was appointed experimentally under a joint finance scheme between the area health authority and the borough (Day and Mogridge, 1981). She was seconded to the social services department, with responsibilities for preventive care, health education and liaison (between health and social services staff), and had a particular responsibility for the elderly and handicapped. This scheme, which is being evaluated, is one where the health visitor is not in a primary health care team. It shows - as do other schemes which will be referred to - that the particular training and skills of health visitors can be utilized in various community settings and not just within the primary health care team.

Day (1983) subsequently visited a small randomly selected sample of persons over 75 years of age to administer a questionnaire relating to their health and social conditions - and also the sort of regular contact if any they would like with health visitors or other providers of health advice. She found that:

Although over half the respondents identified areas with which they required help and
advice, only nine opted for a home visit, but
thirty-one out of the thirty-two opted for a
postal screening questionnaire which would be
sent personally by their own general practitioner.
...Other services such as a clinic, a
telephone call from the health visitor, media
coverage of health in local newspapers etc.,
were also preferred to the home visit. It
would appear from this small survey that elderly people preferred to maintain a level of
control over the services they receive opting
for those which do not encroach upon them personally, but remain distant from them.

In a pilot scheme in Manchester, a geriatric
care team is led by a health visitor (Halladay,
1981). The health visitor liaises between hospitals, community health services and social services, taking case referrals from these. The team
provides support and nursing help for the elderly
and aims to keep people in their own homes as far
as possible. The funding for this scheme came from
'inner-city' money.

A scheme at Kidderminster provides for a geriatric liaison health visitor leading a team to
give continuing care for patients discharged from
hospital (Thursfield, 1979). The liaison health
visitor is assisted by two SRNs with district nursing qualifications who in turn act as team leaders
to 'clinical assistants' who are SRNs each attached
to one general practice. The geriatric liaison
health visitor is notified of admissions so that
the home conditions of the elderly patient can be
assessed by someone in the team. The information
from this assessment is included in hospital case
notes. Each patient is visited on discharge and
also all known elderly are visited routinely by the
'clinical assistants'. The liaison between hospital and community care which the scheme provides
aims to give support to patients, to check on their
progress, and avoid duplication of visits by professional staff.

Victor and Vetter (1985) carried out a study
showing that there is a marked increase in the use
of the health visiting service by elderly patients
who have been discharged from hospital. They
report:

123

A four per cent random sample of elderly patients (that is, aged 65 and over) who had been discharged from NHS non-psychiatric hospitals in Wales was interviewed three months after discharge using a postal questionnaire. Data were collected about the social characteristics of patients, their morbidity and contact with the health visiting service. Compared with before admission, contact with health visitors increased five-fold after discharge from hospital.

The health visitors were only seeing a minority of elderly patients after discharge from hospital, those considered to be at 'high risk'. The authors point out that if health visitors routinely visited all elderly patients after discharge and if the discharge rate is increased, there would need to be 'a massive expansion of the service.'

A psychogeriatric liaison health visitor has been attached to a psychogeriatric assessment unit in Southampton (Griffiths and Eastwood, 1974). She liaises with community health and social services about discharged patients, handing over to the community health visitor immediately if the patient is already known to them, or establishing the link if this is missing.

An attempt to evaluate the effect of 'focused health visitor intervention' on a group of elderly women in Scotland was made by Luker (1981, 1982). Using two groups of elderly in a cross over study (see page 190), it was found that up to 43% of health problems did improve with 'intervention' (an effect which lasted for five months), although there was no clear improvement in 'life satisfaction', and not all the cases wanted to continue being visited. The elderly in the study generally saw the health visitor as someone to call in when they were ill or had a particular need, rather than as an agent of preventive health care who could give advice.

Another smaller study was carried out by Lam (1984) 'to evaluate the effectiveness of the health visitor's attendance to a group of 50 elderly on the number of general practitioner visits required by these patients'. The health visitor made an initial assessment visit and follow-up visits were made by an assisting SEN, until a new problem arose – such as hospital treatment – in which case the health visitor would do another assessment visit. Over time, the data suggest 'that the health visitor's attendance seems to reduce the number of general practitioner attendance required by the elderly by as much as 26 per cent over a four-year period.

Vetter et al. (1984) carried out a randomized controlled study in two localities in Wales - Powys (Rural) and Gwent (Urban) - to assess the effectiveness of intervention by health visitors for persons aged over 70 years.

> Independent assessments made at the beginning and end of the study show that the health visitor in an urban practice had some impact on her caseload of patients; she provided more services for them, their mortality was reduced and their quality of life improved, though the last measure just failed to be statistically significant. The health visitor working in a rural practice had no such effect.

The intervention took the following form:

> The health visitors were restricted to making one unsolicited visit a year... They followed-up patients who were in trouble at that visit and they were also alerted by the other professionals in the practice if one of their patients had any difficulties.

The health visitors, who were specially employed for the purpose,

> were instructed to interview patients and to keep notes according to usual health visiting practice. In addition a problem sheet and procedure form had to be completed at each interview. These were copied on to a card which was placed in the patients' practice notes and this acted as a means of communication between the practitioners and the health visitors.

Two health authorities responding to the CNO survey mentioned having liaison health visitor schemes for the elderly. One scheme was for liaison between hospital and community, and in the other, which was joint funded, a health visitor liaised between primary care teams, a day hospital, three sheltered housing schemes, and a geriatric consultant (Bideford, North Devon Health Authority).

Developments in the last decade

Five health authorities reported having auxiliaries or SRNs to help health visitors in visiting the elderly, and a sixth (Worcester and District Health Authority) had taken this a stage
further:

A health visitor, supported by SRNs (Staff
Nurse) and teams of part-time Nursing Auxiliaries, provides health care to frail elderly people in their own homes. In addition
to her health promotion and health education
role, the health visitor identifies simple
health and hygiene needs - for example regular
bathing, hair washing, help with dressing -
which can enable elderly people to maintain
their independence for as long as possible.
Because this team is separate from the Acute
District Nursing Services, the care is not
reduced when the District Nursing Sisters are
under pressure.

Health visitors and family and child health care
Traditionally the health visitor's routine
work has been with babies and mothers, and this
pattern is borne out by the findings of the OPCS
survey (Dunnell and Dobbs, 1982). Most of the time
spent by health visitors in clinics was concerned
with babies and young children (69%), and with parents or expectant parents (10%). On visits, health
visitors spent 62% of their time with children up
to the age of 15. Some developments in this area
of care have been reported.

Experimental evening health education sessions
on early antenatal and pre-conceptual health were
held for intending or expecting parents by health
visitors, in a pilot scheme described by Gillies
and Chaudhry (1984). The eight sessions provided
information and advice on health care before, during, and after, pregnancy; including the dangers of
smoking and alchohol and the need to stop oral contraception well before conception. Over half the
attenders (23 out of 40) responded to a questionnaire and felt the sessions had been worthwhile; a
number said they had made changes in their lifestyle as a result.

Health visitors have also been involved in
intensive home visiting of infants at risk of un-
expected infant death. Studies undertaken in
Sheffield have developed a scoring system for infants at birth to identify infants at risk of un-
expected infant death (Carpenter, 1983, Carpenter

et al. 1983, and Jepson, 1984). Those infants at risk (about 14%) are then visited intensively by health visitors, and a reduction in infant mortality has been directly attributed to the effects of this programme of visiting. In the early years of the study (1973-75) this intensive visiting was done by research health visitors, but since 1975 the responsibility for visiting the high risk infants has been with health visitors in the primary care team. Carpenter et al. conclude that the extra care given to high-risk infants by health visitors accounts for 15% of the reduction in the 'possibly preventable post perinatal mortality rate' during the period of the study (from 1973-79). The authors suggest that 'home visiting by health visitors is highly cost-effective'. The Sheffield scoring system for high risk infants has been tried in other areas of the country, with varying degrees of success. A modified version of the scoring system is being evaluated in Southampton (Harris et al. 1982)

Some informal schemes to help mothers and young children have been described. In one scheme, a health visitor and a psychiatric social worker together ran a group for mothers and babies in a health clinic in London (Thomas and Sullivan, 1983). At the regular informal meetings, the 'professionals' stayed for an hour with the mothers and babies to discuss and advise on any topics or problems the mothers themselves raised. The behaviour of the children at the group provided examples of 'child management' problems to discuss. Another similar scheme is described by Tully et al. (1983):

> A health visitor coordinated a short course held in a child health clinic for a group of 14 parents and their young children. This enabled parents and children to explore a variety of play activities together. The parents made new friends and received health education, and student health visitors had an opportunity to observe children at play and to develop their own group skills.

Moulds et al. (1985) describe two innovations in their primary care team. Firstly they have introduced an appointment system for one of the two weekly well-baby clinics, a system which has been successful, and where mothers see the health visitors individually in a room. Secondly they ran a 'six week postnatal support group for first-time mothers', where baby care is discussed, and mothers are encouraged to get to know each other. It is reported that mothers who attended 'required less health visiting time at well-baby clinics and requested very few house calls'.

A health visitor in South London described how, as a member of a steering committee, she helped initiate the setting-up in 1984 of a family centre, funded by the Urban Aid Scheme (Phillips, 1986). The centre provides a day nursery and is a 'focus of activity for families with young children', and employs ten staff. The health visitor concerned saw her role as 'a 'catalyst' in mobilizing resources within the community' where ill health was caused by social and environmental problems.

A health visitor in Newcastle has described her work in an inner city multi-disciplinary intervention project, working with parents and children (Pearson, 1985). The project began in 1979, and aims to provide 'extra medical and nursing input for children in an inner city area' as well as assisting in the integration of services for children, encouraging families and the community

> to assume a greater share of the responsibility for the health of their children ... to learn more about the needs of children in a disadvantaged area and to develop a community resource for undergraduate and postgraduate training.

The health visitor is one among a multidisciplinary team, and has a caseload, in addition to working with playgroups, parent groups, acting as a resource person, and being involved in training, research, and development. A major implication of the project is that 'each health visitor has a responsibility to identify the needs of the area, to work out appropriate responses to those needs and to establish priorities'.

The work of a specialist health visitor providing a home based service for families with young children is described by Pritchard and Appleton (1986). She works for a hospital based child development centre giving families the option of home based intervention, and visits are made by appointment. A six-month evaluation of the treatment programme for 46 children, using a behaviour screening questionnaire completed by the parents (and in addition a general health questionnaire for parents using the crying baby clinic) showed that the intervention programme was successful.

Initiatives in providing health care for 'travelling families' have been made. In east London a health visitor was appointed in 1981 as a health worker for travellers (Lawrie, 1983). The post is funded by the Inner City Partnership Scheme, and was established through the collaboration of three inner London health authorities. The health worker has recorded contacts with 93 families, to whom general health advice, family planning, some child health clinic facilities and immunization have been offered, at the camp site. Two general practitioners have co-operated in giving this service which has resulted in higher immunization levels for children. The author stresses the importance of health workers going to camp sites in order to provide health services, and if necessary following up families as they move. In Sheffield a health visitor has undertaken to provide health visiting services to travellers' families in addition to her normal caseload (Peck, 1983). The families are encouraged to attend a local clinic, but it is hoped in future to bring a mobile clinic to the sites.

Pahl and Vaile (1986), in their study of environment, health and health care amongst travellers in Kent, used, health visitors in whose areas the travellers' sites were located as interviewers. Among their recommendations were the following: 'Health authorities should appoint a named health visitor or health visitors (not more than two) to be responsible' for keeping updated information on all sites.

In particular environmental conditions on the sites, as well as knowing who is living there with special regard to mothers and children and for making close contacts and for health education. Specialist health visitors in neighbouring districts can more easily keep in contact when Travellers move on. They could also act as advocate for health and health care for Gypsies.

...Health Authorities should design personal case records to be handed to and kept by Gypsy mothers to facilitate continuity of care when moving on.

...Health Authorities should consider the provision of mobile services to seek out clients and provide health care on permanent and unauthorised sites. A mobile clinic (caravan) should be multipurpose and should provide antenatal care, child surveillance and immunization, health education and family planning, cervical cytology and possibly minor treatments.

Ten health authorities responding to the CNO survey referred to schemes in which health visitors were involved in teams in family and child health care. These included schemes providing for case work with families, day centres for the care and assessment of mentally handicapped children, prevention of child abuse, and parentcraft classes for prospective adoptive parents. (See also pages 138-139.)

Health visitors and psycho-social problems

There is evidence that a substantial proportion of health visitors' cases involve a psycho-social content, particularly in households without children under five years. (See e.g. Clark, 1976, who reports this in her study of 2,057 home visits by health visitors in Berkshire in 1969.) The results of a pilot stage of a study (Briscoe and Lindley, 1982) showed that in one week's visiting, a health visitor identified and/or managed two different types of psycho-social problems in routine visits to 17 families. More problems were classified as potential rather than actual, emphasizing the preventive approach of health visiting in this field. Some articles have reported schemes in which the psychological skills of health visitors were developed and used.

Mottram (1980) describes group psychotherapy sessions being held in a practice with nurses or health visitors acting as group leaders together with general practitioners.

A psychiatrist (Clarke, 1980) describes a series of seminars held in a health centre, in which health visitors discussed 'principles of assessment and management' of cases with the psychiatrist. This developed skills in the health visitors, and brought the psychiatrist into contact with the primary health care team.

In Sussex (Reavley, 1981), a clinical psychologist reported on shared clinic sessions held with the health visitors since 1979. Selected patients see the psychologist, who manages these cases to-

gether with the health visitor. The author concludes that:

> Working together has produced a better clin-
> ical service and a more effective use of our
> resources. Good communication about the cases
> ... has been made much easier by having a
> clinic at the same time and in the same place.

A health visitor in Harrow describes how she
helped young mothers to form home-based groups for
mutual support (Hiskins, 1981, 1982). The scheme
has evolved since 1969. Each group of 6-8 mothers
has a 'leader' who is one of the mothers, and they
meet in each other's homes in the area. A 'unit'
is formed by six groups, and 'large social events'
are organized by the 'unit' which includes husbands. There is a monthly newsletter with ideas
and information and a library of relevant books
bought by fund raising. As a result of a study by
interview of five groups of 43 mothers, the author
concludes that the existence of the groups prevents
isolation and helps prevent psychosomatic illness,
as families give mutual support and mothers have
friends to turn to. In this scheme, the health
visitors have facilitated self-help in order to
prevent psycho-social problems developing.
    Another type of self-help group for mutual
support was initiated by a health visitor (Drummond
1984) in collaboration with an Age Concern worker.
The group, which meets in an east London health
centre, consists of carers for elderly relatives.
The carers discuss mutual problems and provide support for each other, with the professionals acting
as facilitators.
    Webb (1985) described the setting up of a
hysterectomy self-help group which offered information and support both before and after the operation to patients and their husbands or partners.
She emphasized the important contribution that a
health visitor had to offer such groups. In subsequent correspondence, Sarson and Allen (1985) and
Vaughan (1985) agreed with this writer on the importance of such groups and drew attention to their
spread throughout the country (at least 22 were
mentioned), but questioned whether the active involvement, at least as an organizer, of a health
visitor or even a nurse was necessary for their
successful functioning.
    Four health authorities responding to the CNO
survey mentioned support for isolated or depressed

mothers, by clubs, support groups, or counselling by health visitors. In another authority a health visitor worked with psychiatric patients in a large rural area, and local support groups had been set up. (See also page 13 6.)

Health visitors liaising between hospital and community services

A variety of health visitor liaison schemes have developed for different groups of patients, and with the health visitor based in either the hospital or in the community.

A number of health visitor liaison schemes were investigated by Paxton (1974). The author found paediatric, maternity, geriatric, diabetic, orthopaedic and chest clinic health visitors liaising between hospital and community, and one between hospital and school for physically and mentally handicapped children. It was concluded that although liaison schemes were costly, the benefits to patients - as reported by staff - must be taken into account. The benefits included continuity of care, speedy transmission of information and better staff relationships.

Three schemes whereby a health visitor liaises between hospital and community in relation to elderly patients, are referred to in the section of this book on 'Health visitors and the elderly' - page 11 8 (Halladay, 1981, Griffiths and Eastwood, 1974 and Thursfield, 1979). Some schemes relating to other groups of patients are described below.

In Leeds, a scheme operates whereby two health visitors are attached to the rehabilitation team in a hospital (Firth et al. 1978). The health visitors, in addition to their normal duties, accompany the rehabilitation team on ward rounds and follow up patients in the community after discharge. An assessment of the home conditions is made, if necessary, by the health visitor before discharge, and she provides support during the critical first week after discharge from hospital. This support includes liaison with the general practitioner, ensuring voluntary bodies and social services undertake services agreed and advising the patient and family on self-care at home. The patient is handed over to the usual health visitor when the patient is stabilized at home. The scheme was studied for its effect upon patients and it was concluded that it resulted in a lower re-admission rate.

A liaison health visitor works with an oncology outpatients department in Glasgow (Trotter et al. 1981). The health visitor 'gathers information about patients, relatives, and their problems, ... co-ordinates the provision of support services, and... is a counsellor'. By visiting patients in their homes she is able to uncover problems, e.g. of pain control, which patients find more difficult to raise in the ward or clinic. She is hospital-based and may visit patients without consulting the general practitioner first. Her work has been studied and it was concluded that she is 'an essential part of the oncology team'.

An example of diabetic liaison health visitors, based in the community but liaising with the hospital team, is found in Leeds (Jackson, 1979). In this instance one health visitor works full-time with diabetic patients, while another still retains some normal health visiting caseload. It is felt that the scheme has enabled patients to be more often stabilized at home, or to spend less time in the ward for stabilization.

In Leicester a paediatric liaison health visitor has been long established, since 1968 (Matheson and Tillson, 1978). She liaises between wards, out-patients and the home, supervising home nursing of ill children and giving advice to parents. It was felt that the health visitor's work there reduced out-patient visits and saved hospital beds.

Wallis (1982) described her work as a maternity and paediatric liaison health visitor. She visits paediatric and maternity wards and attends the relevant out-patient clinics, talking to staff and patients and passing on all relevant information to family health visitors. Based in a health centre, her time is entirely taken up with gathering and disseminating information.

Two examples of paediatric and maternity liaison health visitors based in hospitals have been described in some detail. One of these is based at the West Middlesex, although she is funded from the community nursing establishment (Ilett, 1984). She visits paediatric, ante and post-natal wards, and other wards or departments where patients in these areas may be found, for instance gynaecology wards, casualty and psychiatric units. From her visits to patients, and attendance at ward rounds she is able to provide a more complete picture of the patient's situation for the relevant community health visitor who takes over at the patient's discharge.

Another liaison health visitor based at a hospital and concerned with paediatric and maternity cases has described an evaluation of her work at University College Hospital, London (Tuplin, 1984). Questionnaires were sent to ward sisters and community health visitors, referrals to community health visitors were monitored over a four month period, and the liaison health visitor kept an activity diary during the same period. Some problems, such as inaccurate or insufficient information being given, were identified, but almost all the health visitors and ward sisters thought that the liaison service was useful.

In Preston a system operates whereby family health visitors are informed of any children up to five who have visited an accident and emergency department after an accident, so that the health visitor can go to the home and give advice on safety (Ahamed, 1978, 1982). The information obtained over time has demonstrated the advice on safety most needed at the different ages of children, and it is hoped that in the long term home accidents will be reduced.

Eight health authorities responding to the CNO survey mentioned health visitor liaison schemes in a range of specialities, including diabetic, maternity, paediatric, oncology and psychiatry.

Specialization in health visiting

Currently health visitors tend to be 'specialized' in the care of babies and young children, although they have a wider responsibility for preventive health care generally. There are some advocates of 'specialized' health visitors as such, and examples of a few types of specialized health visitors were found, apart from the 'liaison' and other health visitors with specialist training described in the preceding sections.

One type of specialism advocated is for handicapped children. In Lancaster health district, five health visitors were trained in the Portage system in order to study the effectiveness of providing such a service (Holland, 1981). Each health visitor visited one family with a developmentally delayed child and after six months the service was evaluated. It was found that the health visitors had been able to acquire the skills necessary to provide the service, and they had been able to continue normal duties as well. The children had progressed and the parents were enthusiastic.

A study of specialized health visitors working with Down's syndrome infants by Cunningham et al. (1982a) is summarized by them as follows:

A health visitor was seconded to a university based research team studying early intervention with families who have an infant with Down's syndrome. She was given a three week practical training and then provided a home-based service for 61 families, visiting every 6 weeks until 2 years of age. Infant development and parental satisfaction with the service were compared to previous findings of the research group. Parental satisfaction was found to be very high and the progress of the infants compared favourably to previous studies. Following this, two field health visitors were given the training and then provided a service in their local area. The progress of the infants was monitored at 6-month intervals until 2 years of age, and parents were interviewed. Again no difference was found in the developmental progress of the infants and previous groups and parental satisfaction was high.'

The importance of early intervention is stressed by the authors, who found that the short course of practical training for the health visitors involved was adequate for children up to 18 months, when more specialized training is needed to provide help for these children. The health visitors in the study were not carrying normal caseloads as well: however, the authors report that several family health visitors had said they would prefer to visit the Down's syndrome children themselves and that family health visitors

often maintained a joint service with the specialist health visitor. Where this has happened, the comments of the parents, the family health visitor and the specialist health visitor strongly suggest that it is the most satisfactory approach.

However, in a later article (Cunningham et al. 1982b) the same authors report that where the family health visitor (rather than the research health visitor) undertook a 'home visiting intervention programme' with Down's syndrome infants, the results were less satisfactory. Although parents took their children more frequently to child health clinics, the health visitors reduced their home visiting rate after the babies were six months, and mothers' satisfaction with the health visiting ser-

135

vice was mixed. Just over half the mothers were positive about the service, but a quarter were indifferent and a fifth were 'hostile'. Some of the problems appeared to arise from conflicting expectations held by the health visitors and the mothers about the role of the health visitor. The authors report that the provision of

> short in-service training courses focusing on practical aspects of early development and stimulation of handicapped infants has resulted in high rates of visiting and parental satisfaction

and such training for family health visitors is recommended.

Specialist health visitors for mentally and physically handicapped children are employed in health districts in Leicestershire (Baker et al. 1980). The health visitors liaise with the senior medical officers, special schools, and social services; and aim 'to provide practical and supportive help to families', 'to develop up-to-date knowledge of all existing services for handicapped children', and 'to give guidance to professional colleagues'.

There is an example of a scheme involving a specialist health visitor with the disabled in Southampton (Dawson, 1979), where she is employed in establishing and maintaining a 'register of dependent disabled adults' (up to 65 years). Detailed information about the disabled person, their family and circumstances, is obtained, and this is updated once every six months or more often if the situation is deteriorating. The names of persons who could be on the register are obtained from the general practitioners. It was hoped that by using the information, the health visitor could provide a supportive service to these persons and their families, foresee impending crises and avert them, thus maintaining persons in the community if possible.

The work of a specialist health visitor in a community psychiatric unit is described by Houseman et al. (1981). The unit is staffed by a team of professionals and volunteers, the health visitor being concerned with family work in particular. She holds 'an open, "walk-in" clinic which offers clients the opportunity to refer themselves', and may call on the help of other unit staff in the treatment of clients. The authors conclude that

the health visitor has a developing role in an open
community psychiatric unit.

Finally there are some schemes described where
the health visitor is concerned with oncology patients and the care of the dying. A system in Edinburgh in which hospital-based health visitors contribute to 'the support and care of terminally ill
patients and their relatives' was described by
Murray et al. (1974). The patients were those attending a hospital respiratory disease unit for
bronchial carcinoma. The health visitors in this
scheme were geographically deployed, based at the
hospital, and worked with the consultant physician.
They visited patients regularly, obtaining information about social and economic conditions, and giving support and advice to the patient and his family before and after his death. It was felt that
this support helped families to manage nursing by
themselves without necessarily involving district
nurses, and enabled patients to avoid going back
into hospital.

In Brent, the health district employs a health
visitor and an oncology nurse to give support and
advice (not practical nursing) to patients who were
dying and to their families (Wilshaw and Aplin,
1981). Most referrals came from consultants, but
general practitioners, district nurses, social workers and health visitors also refer. The service
provides counselling for patients and relatives,
and bereavement counselling after death.

(The appointment of a health visitor to work
with travellers' families has been referred to in
the section above on 'Health visitors and family
and child health care', page 129.)

Of the eleven health authorities responding to
the CNO survey who mentioned having schemes involving specialist health visitors, nine of these were
for mentally handicapped children and in some cases
also for physically handicapped children. Of the
other two authorities, one authority reported having a specialist diabetic health visitor and the
other had appointed two NNEBs* responsible to a
health visitor to

> visit inadequate or culturally disadvantaged
> families on a regular basis to reinforce ad-
> vice given by health visitors and support
> mothers with premature or handicapped babies.

*i.e. Staff possessing the Nursery Nurses Exami-
nation Board's qualification.

They extend the range of simple play opportunities for children in the home and clinics.

Health visitors and screening, surveillance and
assessment (other than for the elderly)
    Health visitors by definition are concerned
with the prevention of ill-health and its early
detection. This is particularly so in the work of
the health visitor with babies and young children,
the age group with which the health visitor is most
concerned, and some studies in this field are described below. Health visitors are also involved in
schemes to screen adult age groups, and some of
these are also described. (Where health visitors
have taken part in schemes to screen for ill-health
among the elderly, these schemes are described in
the section on 'Health visitors and the elderly'.)

a)   Health visitors and the screening of infants
and children. One Scottish study in a health board
addressed itself to the problem of 'who should
carry out developmental screening examinations?'
(Lawrence and Sklaroff, 1978). Using the same developmental screening record, one group of young
children were examined by general practitioners and
health visitors, a second group by medical officers
and health visitors, and a third group by health
visitors alone. It was concluded that health visitors could use the screening record satisfactorily,
in both clinic and home settings, although health
visitors tended to take longer than the doctors to
complete the test.
    In another Scottish study, health visitors,
supervised by clinical medical officers, undertook
neurodevelopmental screening of infants in a health
district (Morris and Hird, 1981). The authors concluded that this method of screening was practical,
and that

        the percentage of children identified as
        requiring further investigation in the present
        cross sectional study compares favourably with
        other more doctor-orientated schemes,

although they considered a longitudinal study was
necessary to corroborate these findings.
    Again in Scotland, a study was carried out

        to test the feasibility of a standard pro-
        gramme of preschool developmental screening,

where children were screened at six weeks,
eight months, 18 months and three years

(Berkeley et al. 1984). The health visitors and
general practitioners taking part were given special training and together with clinical medical
officers carried out the screening programme, except that the health visitors did not do physical
examinations. The authors conclude that such a
screening programme is feasible, although it takes
quite a lot of time. They suggest that health
visitors could take on 'the main burden of the
screening programme'.

In a postal enquiry which obtained information
from 88 out of 90 AHAs about their policies on
child health surveillance, wide variations were
found (Connolly, 1982). Areas varied in the degree
of health visitor involvement and in the assessment
criteria used. A small sample of health visitors
questioned as part of the same study also showed
some disagreement about assessment criteria, and it
was reported 'that regardless of the AHA child
health assessment policy, health visitors made
their own evaluations of childrens' well-being'.
The author recommends that each region should set
up a working party 'to examine the health visitors'
work in child assessment to identify where they can
most effectively contribute in this work'.

Five health authorities responding to the CNO
survey said they had instituted developmental clinics for children, with health visitors collaborat-
ing with doctors and other |professionals in the
assessments. In one authority (Hull), an orthop-
tist screened young children for visual defects,
two authorities had schemes to identify children at
risk from abuse, and in another (Portsmouth and
south east Hampshire) health visitors undertook a
programme of visits to families at risk of Sudden
Infant Death when scored according to the Sheffield
system.

b) Health visitors and the screening of adults.
One health visitor has described her work in a
well-woman centre in London (Newell, 1984). The
centre opens once a week, and as well as the usual
screening procedures (cervical smears, breast
examination etc.) provides a marriage guidance
counsellor and referral to other agencies and
promotes discussion and self-help groups for women.

The idea of 'well-woman' clinics is well established, and now the idea of 'well-man' clinics

seems to be taking hold. Three articles describe
clinics for men, although there is variation in the
age groups which the clinics are intended to
screen. A clinic in Devon held by a health visitor
offers screening for all men aged 40 to 60 registered in two practices. Attenders have blood pressure taken and urinalysis done, as well as a general discussion of health problems (Austin, 1984).
A clinic in West Sussex run by a health visitor and
community sister aims to screen men registered in
their practice, aged 35 to 65 years (Carroll-
Williams and Allen, 1984) and provides a similar
service to the Devon clinic. In Glasgow, two male
health visitors have also set up a pilot 'well-man'
clinic, aimed at men aged 20 to 50, and described
by a visiting journalist (Sadler, 1985). Attenders
have blood pressure, urine, lung function, eyesight
and hearing checked, complete a detailed questionnaire, and receive advice and counselling in a
lengthy session with a health visitor.

The two health visitors were subsequently
appointed to run the 'Goodhearted Glasgow' campaign
of the Greater Glasgow Health Board - a cardiovas-
cular disease prevention programme. The goal of
this campaign was 'to reduce the number of cases of
coronary heart disease and stroke in Glasgow by 10%
over the next ten years'. (Quotation from handout
(undated) headed 'Goodhearted Glasgow', issued by
Greater Glasgow Health Board.) This involved cam-
paigns in the media and via schools etc. relating
to diet and lifestyle, and screening via primary
health care teams. These teams would also inform
and advise the public and treat as necessary using
standardized guidance and methods of treatment
(provided in the form of a manual as part of the
project to family doctors and district nurses and
health visitors).

One scheme aiming at prevention of diseases in
later life was set up in South Hammersmith. Those
over 50 were invited to come to clinics run by a
health visitor and a clinic nurse, for some screening and health advice (Figgins, 1979). This of
course was not within a general practice context,
but the clinic was in an area with many single-
handed general practitioners where presumably it
would be more difficult to set up this type of
clinic within general practice.

In another scheme the attached health visitor
played a role in a feasibility study in Scotland
which was set up to see if men could be screened
for risk of coronary heart disease and would take

advice to reduce the risk factors (Rankin et al. 1976). Men aged 35-44 were invited to contact the health visitor, who gave advice on diet, exercise and smoking, and she arranged for an examination and tests by the general practitioner at which she assisted. At a follow-up of the men some months later, tests showed an improvement (e.g. in weight, plasma chloresterol etc.) and the men claimed that they had increased exercise taken and reduced smoking. It was concluded that advice could change habits, and that this scheme is feasible in a general practice with attached health visitors.

A health visitor in South Wales has reported on her involvement in a hypertension clinic in general practice (Jones, 1984). Patients of the practice who have been found to be hypertensive regularly attend the clinic where they see the general practitioner and the health visitor, having routine checks and receiving advice on such matters as diet, smoking and exercise.

Seven health authorities in the CNO survey reported holding 'well-woman' type clinics, and one of these, plus two other authorities, also reported holding 'well-man' clinics.

DISTRICT NURSING

Organizational aspects of district nursing
The organization of district nursing, unlike that of health visiting where the issue of attachment versus geographical deployment is still debated, is not a subject which has produced a similar controversy in the literature.

The study by Poulton (1977), to which we have already referred regarding health visitors (see page 114) concluded in the case of district nurses that:

> The home nurse also shows a significant variation of working patterns between schemes throughout almost all aspects of her work. The main differences are:
> 1. The attached nurse spends less time on visiting patients at home but compensates for it by carrying out care at the surgery.
> 2. The aligned nurse and nurses engaged on relief work, spend more time on travelling than their colleagues.

Developments in the last decade

The West Midlands Regional Health Authority,
Management Services Division (1977) reported on a
study of attachment versus geographical allocation
in the Salop Area Health Authority for district
nurses. In this study the alternative methods of
organization considered were compared with respect
to attitudes of district nurses and general practitioners and to costs. Costs of the alternatives
were examined via a simulation study. In particular, theoretical models of what was meant by
attachment and geographical allocation were constructed incorporating certain highly specific
assumptions. These models were then applied to the
data on the work of district nurses for two areas,
(Shrewsbury and Telford), which had been collected
at an earlier phase of the investigation in order
to compare the different travelling times and costs
involved in adopting the two methods of organizing
district nurses' work to deal with the work patterns as actually recorded in 1976. Where pure
attachment or geographical allocation approaches
were compared using the theoretical model approach,
geographical allocation emerged as considerably
cheaper than attachment. However, the point was
made that in practice the schemes adopted were
mixed rather than pure attachment or pure geographical allocation making it difficult on the
basis of simply collecting data about them to infer
precisely the impact of one approach or the other.
Equally of course the idealized versions of attachment and geographical allocation encapsulated within the theoretical models may not ever exist in
practice.

Four health authorities responding to the CNO
survey mentioned that their district nurses were
attached to GP practices, in three authorities
district nurses were mentioned as being aligned
with general practitioners but visited patients
within a geographical area, and one authority reported that it had gone back to a geographical
system entirely. West Lambeth Health Authority
(London) reported that they had negotiated with a
neighbouring authority (Camberwell) that district
nurses would cover all general practice patients,
whichever authority the patients lived in.

District nurses providing services out of normal
hours
Several schemes for providing night nursing or
night sitting services, which are becoming widespread, were reported on in the literature. These

142

schemes need to be seen in the context of the major national (England and Wales) survey undertaken by Harrisson et al. (1983) of evening, night and early morning (district nursing and related) services. It was found that of the 151 districts who responded in the 'main study' (stage one) only two did not have some form of out-of-hours service - though it is possible that among the non-responding districts, a higher proportion may not have had such services. In 13% of those districts (respondents) which did provide an out-of-hours service, the service was offered 'in parts of the district only'. The majority of districts (83% of respondents) recruited staff especially for out-of-hours work but the remaining 17% offered a day staff 'on-call' system of some kind. The authors noted

> that costs were particularly high in Districts operating full 24 hour nursing services. Some Districts chose the low cost alternative of day nurses working on-call outside normal hours but it was shown that out-of-hours services operated in this way were less extensive in the range of skills and services provided than those for which staff were specially employed and also had disadvantages for the nurses concerned. The cost of evening services tended to be high because the majority of districts staffed them with specially employed nurses.

Among respondents it was found that 98% of districts which provided out-of-hours services, 'employed state registered nurses, 46% employed state enrolled nurses and 69% employed nursing auxiliaries'. It was also noted that a substantial amount of non-technical care was carried out and many NHS staff suggested that more untrained staff should be employed, although it was recognized that not all out-of-hours work falls neatly into technical and non-technical categories.
In the districts responding to the enquiries of Harrisson et al. (1983),

> the most common types of out-of-hours care provided were: general nursing care for the highly dependent (98% of districts), injection service (97%), putting patients back to bed (92%), emergency requests (unspecified) from existing patients (90%).

In a survey of the opinions of samples of general practitioners and district nurses which also formed part of Harrisson et al. (1983), night sitting services were found to be held in

> high regard by nurses and general practi-
> tioners for providing continuity of care and
> reducing workload. Such services because of
> their flexibility are able to respond to local
> need when required .... although close liaison
> between health and social services depart-
> ments, which exists in many districts, would
> be essential. Just over 40% of the responding
> general practitioners and district nurses
> practised in districts in which the social
> services department provided a night sitting
> service.

Out-of-hours nursing services then are an extension of community nursing provision, being under
the direction of community nursing officers. The
staff of them are usually recruited in addition to
the day community nursing staff and are paid for
from health authority funds or joint health and
social service funds, in one instance reported
below. Nursing of patients dying from cancer is
undertaken from charitably funded Marie Curie
nurses but where not enough of these nurses were
available, the night nursing services provided an
alternative. Some examples of these schemes are
described below.
In a scheme in Fife there is a service for
short term cases, e.g. care of the dying, or for
longer term cases but less intensively, e.g. one or
two nights a week to relieve relatives. Patients
are referred by general practitioners or district
nurses and cases are allocated by the nursing
officer (Gillespie, 1980). Fife also provides a
'tucking down' service for patients needing longer
term care. One nurse can visit several patients in
an evening to do this, whereas with the night nursing service one nurse is with the patient all
night. Generally the nurses felt the scheme worked
well, and although there was no proof, it was felt
that these services kept patients at home and out
of hospital for longer than would otherwise be the
case. However, the one-to-one ratio of night nursing is expensive, compared to the 'tucking down'
service.
Aberdeen provides a night nursing service
(Jack, 1976) and also evening visits to psycho-

geriatric patients. Nurses from the psychiatric hospital visit patients referred to them by staff from the psychogeriatric day hospital, aiming to delay or prevent in-patient admissions.

In Lancaster a pilot scheme for night nursing was described by Hornby (1976). Day staff were already operating a rota scheme for night emergencies, and to relieve them of this work, two groups of extra part-time nursing staff were recruited. One group dealt with general nursing care, the other group with emergencies at night on a peripatetic basis. It was concluded that the need for, and possibility of, a 24-hour service had been demonstrated. The service provided care for patients waiting for admission to hospital, and it was said that bed usage improved. An unforeseen need was for a night psychiatric service, to support relatives of dying patients, and it was felt that this would be valuable if it could be provided.

A study of the night and evening nursing services in Newham (Martin and Ishino, 1981) concludes that the costs of the services are less than hospital care and enabled patients to remain at home who would otherwise go into hospital and block beds. Patients for the night and evening services are referred by general practitioners, community nurses, hospital consultants and casualty departments. No study of quality of care was undertaken, although it was reported that patients were pleased to be at home still. The study estimated that only care in Part III accommodation* was less costly than intensive home care, but the patients were too ill or handicapped to qualify for Part III homes.

A night nursing service in Southend (Sims, 1981 and 1982) reports that patients seem to have been kept at home rather than being taken into hospital care. Referrals came mainly from the community nursing services, general practitioners and the accident centre.

Another variation on the night nursing services is operated in Rochdale (Anon. 1981). As the night nursing service is limited because of resources, a night sitting service is provided, the sitters being employees of the local authority. The night sitters are usually unqualified and given training by the district nursing staff who also are involved in appointing them. The sitters are sup-

---

*Accommodation provided for the elderly by local authorities under Part III of the National Assistance Act, 1948).

ervised and managed by the district nursing staff. They enabled the night nursing service to be extended, and they stay with patients in the night, with the night nurse visiting the home during that time.

Out-of-hours district nursing services were widely reported in the CNO survey. Altogether 38 authorities referred to providing services out-of-hours, and as in the literature these services ranged from evening or 'tucking down' schemes through to night sitting and 24-hour nursing services.

District nurses and the elderly

Care of the elderly forms a substantial proportion of the district nurse's work, and with an increasing proportion of the population coming into this group the demand on the nurse is increasing. In 1983 45% of cases attended by district nurses were to those of 65 or more (Central Statistical Office, 1985) and a survey by the OPCS (Dunnell and Dobbs, 1982) showed that 75% of the district nurses' time was spent with patients over 65. In addition a study by Victor and Vetter (1984) showed that for patients aged 65 years and over, visits from the district nurse increased threefold in the period after discharge from hospital compared to the period before, and that demand for the district nursing services came most from those least able to perform daily living activities.

The services of the district nurse become all the more important given the policy of keeping people at home in the community for as long as possible, and the shortage of beds for the elderly sick. Two studies on this problem give conflicting views on the economic cost of keeping the elderly sick at home. Opit (1977) estimated the cost of caring for a group of elderly sick who were receiving district nurse care. When nursing, home help and social worker times were added to equipment, laundry, meals and social security payments, he concluded that the cost of keeping these patients at home was comparable to keeping them in residential care. An even more serious consideration was the quality of care received by these patients. No objective assessment was available, but the district nurses estimated that nearly 30% of the patients at home were 'receiving either inadequate or inappropriate care'. Maintaining a satisfactory level of care (which may not be possible at home anyway for seriously disabled patients) requires more finance. Opit concludes that without this increase in funding then 'domiciliary care for the elderly sick will be increasingly "economic" simply because the level of care provided becomes increasingly inadequate'.

On the other hand Gibbins et al. (1982) in Cleveland describe a scheme where 'augmented home nursing' was used as an alternative to hospital care for chronic elderly invalids. Extra nursing and home help staff were recruited to provide extra care until, if possible, patients could be referred back to the usual, not 'augmented', level of service provided by district nursing staff and home helps. Gibbins et al. argue that the costs of this are comparable to long-stay care, however they did not take into account the range of costs considered by Opit above.

A pilot study of 'augmented' home care for acutely or sub-acutely ill elderly patients was undertaken in Edinburgh (Currie et al. 1980). Intensive community nursing and medical care (daily visits by a general practitioner or a geriatrician) were given to patients during an acute illness to avoid admission to hospital, and patients' recovery was assessed by tests of function in daily living. The results suggested that recovery was quicker at home than it would have been in hospital, and that the scheme was acceptable to the patients.

A scheme in Norfolk (Allibone, 1979) to provide care for the elderly in the community has involved local people as well as professionals. Apart from 'social' type services, such as transport, a luncheon club and social activities, the scheme also provides a volunteer nursing service, working to help the district nurse. The people providing this service do not necessarily have any nursing experience, so they are given some basic training in home nursing, and carry out for instance bathing and foot care, bed making and some night sitting. The volunteer group have a trained nurse as their 'leader' who liaises with the district nurse about allocation of work. Of course the success of such a scheme depends on having people locally available and willing to do the work and is no substitute for trained nursing care. However, in reports of a research study into this scheme (Allibone and Coles, 1982 and 1984), it was stated that the work of the volunteer nurses reduced by half the number of visits made by community nurses compared with similar areas where there was no volunteer service, and that professionals and volunteers could work together in harmony.

Developments in the last decade

A joint care funded scheme for the elderly in East Sussex (Anon. 1981) provides health services, sheltered housing and Part III accommodation in purpose-built premises. The scheme brings the relevant professionals together on one site where the elderly can go for counselling, social activities and treatment. The scheme provides for an extra district nurse in the locality, so that the extra nurse time needed for the project can be allocated. The nurse is not acting in a new role here so much as in a different structure, involving much closer collaboration - if the scheme works out as the planners hope - between staff in health, housing and social services departments.

Four studies have reported on the use of district nurses doing routine assessments of the elderly. One study in Scotland (Wallace, 1975) reported on a general practice where the district nursing sister routinely did assessments of patients of 75 and over. She makes an assessment of their housing conditions, social contacts, mobility, self-care and health. The author feels that although this type of assessment is associated with health visitors, having a nurse visit ensures immediate treatment without delays due to referral. Assessment of the elderly is an area where it is not clear who is most appropriate to undertake it. Wallace reported that the nursing sister aimed to educate the elderly to improve their health, and to detect early signs of abnormality.

In another Scottish study (Barber and Wallis, 1976), district nurses on the Island of Mull, who combine the functions of health visiting and district nursing, undertook assessments of patients aged 75 and over. The nurses completed an assessment record (which had been developed in other studies) which recorded medical and social details about the patient, and 'several areas of problem and unmet need' were found.

A study in Birmingham used nurses (including a research nurse as well as district nurses) to survey the medical and social needs of a sample of the elderly (70 plus) in a general practice. It was concluded that nurses could carry out this kind of screening, and that there was a need for it, judged by the problems which were uncovered (Shaw, 1975). However, these results raised the problem of how to undertake this work, given the manpower which was needed to go out and interview persons in their homes. The practice list was found to be inadequate as a basis for a survey, which required 'a total population register' so that all the elderly in a given geographical area could be contacted. Attachment schemes did not ensure that all the population groups were fully listed.

Gooding et al. (1982) describe a scheme where a nurse visitor was employed part-time in a practice to visit patients of 75 years and over to undertake preventive visiting. She asked patients about their general health and mental state and provided some type of service for 81% of the 282 patients visited in one year. Little unknown major pathology was found, but the nurse visitor provided support for relatives and friends, helped in improving safety and conditions in homes, and tried to help in cases of loneliness. It was hoped that the preventive visiting would have some effect on the use of geriatric beds. So far this had not resulted but the study is continuing.

Authorities responding to the CNO survey reported a variety of schemes developed to improve care for the elderly. Some of these were schemes of a type referred to already in the literature, for example in nine authorities district nurses were involved in screening or surveillance of the elderly and two authorities in Manchester had set up geriatric nursing teams to provide intensive nursing care for the elderly.

In six authorities district nurses were mentioned as undertaking nursing care in residential homes for the elderly. (In some authorities, nursing staff did not nurse patients in residential homes themselves, but gave advice to care staff - this type of scheme is referred to in the section below on 'Nursing and related care - joint schemes with social services', page 156). Six authorities reported district nurses appointed to liaise between hospital and community services, two authorities had appointed district nurses as geriatric visitors, and in Sutton Coldfield district nurses, in consultation with general practitioners, arranged admission of patients to a short stay unit in a small hospital.

Paediatric home nursing

A scheme 'to provide specialized nursing care for sick children in their own homes' has operated in Gateshead since 1974 (Hally et al. 1977). The nursing care is provided by district nurses recruited from the existing general practitioners' attached nursing staff who were given training on the paediatric wards. Children enter the scheme either after discharge from hospital (when they come under the care of the general practitioner) or if requested by the general practitioner, in order to avoid admission to hospital. The scheme enabled children either to avoid admission or reduce their length of hospital stay, which quite apart from reducing pressure on hospital beds, was considered better for the children emotionally. Most of the mothers, who were questioned about their attitudes to the scheme, were satisfied with it.

Atwell (1975) in Southampton, describes paediatric day-case surgery which began there in 1969. Patients are cared for at home by a paediatric home nursing service, formed from district nurses who come on the weekly ward rounds and visit the hospital daily.

A later article about the scheme (Gow and Atwell 1980) describes the further development of the paediatric nursing role. The nurses in the scheme 'are all district nurses with the additional qualification of the registered sick children's nurse', and they work in geographical areas. The paediatric home nurses have several function. These include post-operative care of children admitted for day surgery, the nurse having the right to re-admit a patient if she feels it necessary; care of children discharged early after surgery; help with care of physically handicapped and mentally handicapped; regular medical treatment such as diabetes management or regular injections for certain conditions; care of dying children; and care of children at home for some conditions which would otherwise need hospital admission. The paediatric home nurses are also involved in nurse training in the community, and liaise between hospital and community health services.

A further article on the Southampton scheme by the same authors (Atwell and Gow, 1985) gives some data on the numbers and types of day-surgery operations carried out, and home visits made, using the scheme. From an analysis of the costs of the scheme, based on 1983 figures, the authors conclude that substantial savings can be made if some inpatient beds are closed, or if productivity is increased because of earlier discharge to home.

Three health authorities in the CNO survey reported having successful paediatric home nursing schemes including the two, Southampton and Gateshead, which have been written about above, and in addition Brent authority ran such a scheme. A fourth authority reported that their paediatric care team had failed because of 'lack of commitment from paediatricians and general practitioners to maintain children at home'.

Day surgery and early discharge

Day surgery and early discharge schemes have been adopted by hospitals in a number of areas and have a consequent effect upon community nursing services. Several articles described schemes where district nurses looked after day-surgery or early discharge cases. (A scheme for day surgery for children is described in the preceding section.)

A scheme in Bedfordshire is described by Shepherd (1976) in which hernia patients are discharged 48 hours post-operatively. The district nurse visited the home pre-operatively to assess the feasibility of early discharge, and visited after surgery, undertaking removal of sutures. It was said that this system reduced the waiting time for hernia repairs from up to a year down to six weeks.

In Kingston and Richmond Area Health Authority, a district nursing sister (Hart, 1982) has described the way community nursing staff manage day-surgery cases of hernias and varicose vein stripping. Nurses visit the patients preoperatively to check their condition (temperature, pulse, respiration, blood pressure), to give advice, and to assess the facilities in the home. If these facilities are not suitable, despite what the patient has previously said, the nurse will notify the hospital and the patient is referred for normal hospital surgery. The nurses routinely visit twice post-operatively, but may visit or be called for again.

Russell et al. (1977), in Stockton-on-Tees, reported on day surgery for hernias and haemorrhoids, concluding that it is clinically and socially acceptable for patients. However, day patients received 4.18 more visits from district nurses than patients kept in the normal length of time following surgery for these conditions. The general practitioners gave day patients 0.50 more consultations than 'longer stay' patients, so the extra work fell mainly on district nurses.

Ruckley et al. (1978) compared systems of after-care for groups of patients who had had varicose veins or hernia operations. One group was managed in an acute ward post-operatively, another in a convalescent hospital and the third group at home in the care of the general practitioner and district nurse. Most post-operative complications were minor, and for the day-surgery group, the district nurse managed most of these, the general practitioner the remainder. It was found (Prescott et al. 1978) that the day-care system required an average of eight minutes more (including travelling time) per patient for the general practitioner than the other systems did. For the district nurse, the day-care system required over 120 minutes extra time per patient than the other systems. The authors report (Garraway et al. 1978) that patients liked the day surgery system more than the alternatives considered and that caring persons (usually relatives) surveyed did not suggest any major criticisms or disadvantages of this approach and that nurses were able to undertake tasks currently done by doctors. As in the study by Russell et al. referred to above, the extra work with patients resulting from day surgery fell on the district nurses rather than the general practitioners.

In a later article, Ruckley et al. (1980) in Edinburgh describe a survey of the views of district nurses caring for day-surgery patients who had had hernia and varicose vein operations. The nurses reported few problems in post-operative care, and felt the system was better for the patients. Most nurses found the scheme satisfying although it did involve extra work.

By contrast, in one study of orthopaedic short-stay surgery cases (Haines and Thompson, 1982), the authors report that the system of overnight stay and discharge home for patients after surgery did not produce significant workload for district nurses. They state that:

> The district nurses are rarely needed because most operation sites are in dressings that do not need changing. If we consider that the services of the district nurse will be needed for social reasons, we treat these cases as in-patients.

Only one authority responding to the CNO survey mentioned their scheme for district nurses managing day surgery cases - Richmond, Twickenham and Roehampton - which has been referred to above.

District nurses in the treatment room
One trend in the work of the district nurse has been for an increasing proportion of 'first treatments' to be given by them at surgery premises, as opposed to patients' homes. Reedy et al.

(1980) quotes a figure of 55.2 first treatments
being given by district nurses on surgery premises
in 1976, compared to 40.5 in 1972. In Reedy's
survey comparing the activities of health authority
and practice nurses, it was found that - not surprisingly - health authority nurses spent more time
working at surgery premises where a treatment room
was available. Compared to practice nurses, however, Reedy found that the health authority nurses
were less likely to perform more 'technical' procedures such as venepuncture, and likely to undertake more traditional 'caring' activities. Similar
findings were reported in Cartwright and Anderson's
survey (1981), by Bowling (1981) and by Dunnell and
Dobbs (1982), in the OPCS survey.
    We found hardly any other items written about
the district nurses' work in treatment rooms. Most
of the detailed studies of work in treatment rooms
we found have been of places where the practice
nurse undertook all or almost all the work, and
these are referred to below in the section on practice nurse's work in the treatment room. One small
study (McIntosh, 1979) looked at the work of six
district nurses at surgery premises, and found that
they were doing traditional nursing tasks only.
Nurses who undertook longer sessions, e.g. an af-
ternoon in the treatment room, saw more patients
per week than those nurses who mainly gave treatments in patient's homes or had short sessions at
the surgery premises. This is a more efficient use
of nurses' time but there was a limit apparently to
the number of patients willing to travel to the
surgery for traditional treatments - some were
quite resistant to this.
    Four authorities responding to the CNO survey
mentioned the development of treatment room services provided by district nurses or by health
authority employed nurses. The benefits of this
were said to be the mileage and home visits saved
by nurses, and the effective service given to patients.

Intensive home nursing
    Some schemes have been developed to provide
care at home for patients who might otherwise need
to have the kind of intensive nursing care provided
by a hospital. (Two schemes which are specifically
for the elderly have been described in the earlier
section on 'District nurses and the elderly', page
146. See Currie et al. 1980 and Gibbins et al.
1982.)

Developments in the last decade

A well-publicized development is the 'hospital at home' scheme which has been operating in Peterborough since 1978 (Mowat and Morgan, 1982). The pilot scheme, funded by the Sainsbury Trust and the area health authority for an experimental period provides care for patients of all ages who would otherwise have to go into hospital for a short period. Administration of the staff, such as extra nurses, a social worker, physiotherapist, occupational therapist and patients' aides ('a cross between a nursing auxiliary and a home help') is done by a senior nursing officer. The general practitioner is responsible for clinical management and the district nurse for nursing care - she can call upon the 'bank' of staff in the scheme for help as needed. Twenty-four hour cover is available, although usually less has been needed. The scheme is aimed at patients who need intensive care for a short period, for instance for patients who are dying, fractures, acute infections in the elderly, and strokes. A survey of a small number of the patients and staff involved reported overall satisfaction with the scheme. It was felt that, although comparing costs of home and hospital care was difficult, the scheme provided the cheaper alternative. If adopted more generally, it was suggested that shorter waiting lists and fewer hospital beds could result. A full report of this study, which arrived at essentially the same conclusions was subsequently produced (Peterborough Health Authority, 1983).

A later article on the hospital at home scheme (Williams, 1985) reports that a wider range of cases are now undertaken by the scheme, including patients discharged early after such operations as hysterectomy, nephrectomy, and hip replacement. Funding is provided now by Peterborough District Health Authority and the Sainsbury Trust for the time being, with help from the Hospital at Home Friends' Group. Research to examine the quality of care and effectiveness of the scheme is being funded by the DHSS, but is said by Williams to be proving difficult as it is almost impossible to make direct comparisons between hospital in-patient and hospital at home cases.

In Rugby, a new post of 'supplementary nursing sister (district nursing)' has been established, to provide intensive care to certain high-dependency patients (Roper, 1983). The patients who are referred by the district nurses to the supplementary nursing sisters are mostly those needing terminal care, but patients with such conditions as multiple sclerosis, coronary disease and cardio-vascular disease are also cared for. The aim is to supplement, and not to supplant, the services provided by the primary care team. The supplementary nursing sister is able to spend longer periods of time with patients than are the district nurses, and she assesses nursing and social needs, liaising with other professional staff to provide a complete service.

Another way to provide nursing care to patients without transferring them to a general hospital has been developed at Burford Community Hospital in Oxfordshire (Punton, 1984). Here the district nurses are allowed to refer patients directly to the hospital, if they are in need of 'healing nursing care'. The district nurse refers the case to the senior nurse or the staff support nurse and after 'home assessment and discussion with the district nurse and often the general practitioner, the patient is admitted to a nursing bed'. The district nurse visits the patient daily in hospital, and if she wishes, may remain the patient's primary nurse in the hospital. District nurses also participate in the meetings of the nursing team and the multidisciplinary team in the hospital. The author concludes:

> The advantages we have seen at Burford from our three nursing beds must surely show a need for all district nurses to have access to nursing units.

In the CNO survey, Peterborough Health Authority reported its 'hospital at home' scheme described in the literature above. The only other intensive home nursing schemes reported were those for elderly patients, referred to above in the section on 'District nurses and the elderly', page 146.

District nurses and screening, surveillance and assessment

In the literature, three studies reported on district nurses, and one on a nurse, undertaking assessments of the elderly. These studies have been described in the section on 'District nurses and the elderly' above.

Nine health authorities responding to the CNO survey reported that district nurses were involved in schemes for the assessment and screening of the elderly, and in addition in four authorities district nurses were involved in clinics for screening men and women in younger age groups.

Nursing and related care - joint schemes with social services

Some schemes have been jointly funded by health and social services to provide help to enable patients (or 'clients') to stay in their own homes. (Some other schemes which are jointly funded are referred to in the sections 'Health visitors and the elderly', 'District nurses and the elderly' and 'District nurses providing services out of normal working hours'). The elderly feature largely in these schemes of help but younger people needing support for short or long periods may also be included.

In Oxfordshire a scheme began in 1979 to provide help for the frail elderly (Quelch, 1981). A project team is led by a senior social worker, and includes a district nurse and home-care assistants. Referrals come from health and social services, and are assessed by a project team member to see what help is being given and what deficiencies in help could be rectified. The home-care assistants, 'who combine personal and domestic caring activities for clients', provide help if necessary seven days a week and occasionally overnight, working in shifts. Apart from providing long-term help for the frail elderly, the scheme also provides short-term intensive help to restore elderly people who have suffered some form of 'crisis' (physical, mental or social) to a better level of functioning. The scheme aims to avoid or delay the admission of clients to long-term residential care, and to enable some elderly people to leave residential care and live again in the community.

Experimental schemes, started in 1979, to provide 'care attendants' for young disabled people and financed by the Hampshire Joint Care Planning Team have been described by Lovelock (1981). The care attendants are 'best described as a (paid) relative substitute' who do work similar to that done by a variety of persons including nursing auxiliaries and home helps. Evaluation of the schemes was carried out, and both carers and clients were very satisfied. It is concluded that the service improves quality of life, and helps to delay or even prevent 'entry into residential care' sometimes, and that it might be extended to other groups such as the elderly and mentally handicapped.

Developments in the last decade

A scheme (set up in 1978) providing 'short-term intensive support and practical help to clients within their own homes' in Avon County is described by Dexter (1981). The scheme has been funded by the health authority and the county, and pays for 'home aides who are appointed for their previous experience in one of the caring professions'. They are based in a hospital and provide seven days a week, 24-hour cover, aimed at rehabilitating clients, for instance after discharge from hospital, so that after a short period of support clients can manage with a less intensive amount of care. The elderly have been the main users of the scheme, and the home aides, apart from providing practical and personal care aim also to re-educate, stimulate and motivate clients. The scheme is reported to be successful and funding is continuing.

In Rochdale a 'home-care scheme' has been instituted, which provides 'home-care workers' for patients on their discharge from hospital - usually elderly patients. Referrals are made by hospital social workers, with district nurse liaison officers providing the link with primary care teams (Anon. 1981b). This joint care scheme began in 1977 and has expanded to weekend and evening care and long-term care, having originally been intended to provide short-term intensive care only.

The London Borough of Waltham Forest, Social Services Department (1982) reported on a comprehensive evaluation of the service provided by a home-care team based in West Walthamstow. The bulk of the workforce of this home-care team (besides home helps) comprised home-care assistants. The team was led by a home-care coordinator (at the time of the report, a qualified occupational therapist) supported by assistant co-ordinators and advisory, technical and clerical staff. Home-care assistants undertook all the tasks usually associated with home helps and in addition to this:

> Home Care Assistants wash and bath clients, attend to hair care, assist them in dressing and undressing, getting in and out of bed, assist in the use of the toilet, clean up after episodes of incontinence and provide general rehabilitative training.

The home-care service provided by the home-care assistants was at the time of the evaluation confined to clients aged 75 years or more who satisfied criteria which were described in some detail.

Developments in the last decade

In order to facilitate co-operation between the
health and social services in, among other things,
the identification and care of clients needing
home care, a joint-funded post of community liaison
district nurse was established. The home-care liaison component of this post was calculated at 11½
hours per week, though for a variety of reasons the
post holder spent considerably more time than this
working on home-care matters. Initially it was
assumed that all home-care clients would receive a
joint assessment (that is from social services and
nursing) but, since a substantial minority of clients were found not to have had or currently be
receiving district nursing care, this practice was
not invariably followed, particularly where the
district nursing service had previously not been
involved. From a review of the clients accepted on
to the home-care scheme, it appears that there had
been a

> significant reduction of admissions to Part
> III accommodation..... A marked success had
> been achieved in improving the level of func-
> tioning of individual clients and this could
> be further improved by some additional Adviser
> for Disabled hours.

Also it was found that

> in some situations the nurses have been able
> to reduce their involvement. This is partic-
> ularly true of some of those clients receiving
> Nursing two or three times a week for medical
> reasons and situations where the Nurse is vis-
> iting to supervise medication.

Another example of co-operation between health
and social services is also described for Rochdale.
A geriatric-care team has been set up to 'assist
and improve the care of elderly residents of local
authority homes' (Anon. 1981a). The need has arisen because of the number of residents in Part III
accommodation who now require nursing and medical
care. The geriatric-care team comprises two district trained nurses, who did some further training
in geriatrics. They visit local authority homes
'to train and to advise as consultants in health
care'. Training is directed at the care staff of
the homes, who are social services employees, so
that they can better manage problems such as incontinence, drug effects and confusional states. The

158

geriatric-care team, after an initial training and advisory visit to each home, revisit the home to monitor progress.

However, a study of elderly people in residential homes in a London borough, which found a substantial amount of physical dependency and mental confusion in the residents, concluded that skilled nurses should be employed in the homes, rather than depending on district nurses (Bowling and Bleathman, 1982). Most of the community nurses interviewed in the study felt that homes should have their own skilled nurses, and they did not have positive feelings about the times they had spent in the homes in nursing tasks.

Four health authorities in the CNO survey reported that they had established joint funded schemes to give domiciliary care to the elderly or disabled, and four had schemes in which district nurses gave advice to staff in Part III accommodation about the care of the elderly residents. In two cities (Birmingham and Manchester) nursing sisters were involved in the care of the homeless. In Birmingham the nurses are in a team, including a general practitioner and a social worker, which provides GP consultations, treatments, counselling and advice to attenders at a social services department centre for the homeless and rootless. In Manchester a district nursing sister is attached to local authority hostels for the homeless to work with the general practitioner visiting these hostels.

Support services for community nurses in the care of the dying

Numerous schemes for helping in the care of the dying at home have been developed. A survey of health districts and single district areas in England and Wales, and of social service departments was carried out by Wells (1980) to find out what services they provided for the dying and the bereaved in the community. This revealed a variety of services provided by the National Health Service, social services and voluntary organizations, in particular many night nursing, night sitting, home care and counselling schemes. (These services do not of course necessarily apply only to the dying, and a number of schemes described in the literature are referred to in this report elsewhere in connection with district nursing services and general help for the sick and elderly.)

In addition there are specialist advisory teams based in hospitals and hospices, whose medical and nursing staff can advise community nursing staff and general practitioners on problems which arise in the management of the dying patient, such as pain control and dealing with the unpleasant side effects of drugs.

A survey of services in England, Wales and Scotland for terminal care available in December 1980 was reported on by Lunt and Hillier (1981). In domiciliary services, the survey found 32 home-care advisory teams (both NHS and non-NHS) and eight hospital support teams (two non-NHS) with wide variations between health regions. These teams had almost all developed since 1975. The authors recommended that:

> The regional imbalance in the provision of services should be redressed, particularly for home care teams where inequalities are greatest. Improvements could be achieved if the NHS encouraged the voluntary sector to favour the regions at present worst provided.

They advocate giving priority to home-care teams rather than to more in-patient units.

Two examples of advisory teams, one based in a hospital, the other in a hospice, which occur in the literature, are described below. In both examples the primary care team retains clinical and nursing care of the patient, working with the support of the specialist team.

A 'terminal-care support team' has been set up at St Thomas's Hospital in London and their work is described by Bates et al. (1981). The original team comprised a nursing sister, social worker, two doctors (radiotherapists) and the hospital chaplain, and began seeing patients at the end of 1977. The team offers help in controlling symptoms to the hospital staff caring for the patient and to the general practitioner if the patient is discharged home, and is available at nights and weekends. If the general practitioner agrees, the team can offer advice to him and the community nursing staff involved. It is felt that by referring patients to the team earlier in the course of disease, and having their symptoms therefore better controlled, patients were able to be at home more, thus releasing hospital beds. The demand for the services of the team has grown over three years, and as a result the team has expanded, an outpatient clinic has

started, and the team's work with patients in the
community, including bereavement counselling, has
greatly increased. The authors argue that providing such a team is cheaper than hospice care
(although of course patients may occupy beds in
hospital), has teaching potential, and 'can bring
the principles of hospice care to patients at home
and in the hospital'.

An advisory service on terminal care based at
a hospice is described by Doyle (1980 and 1982).
The service operates from a hospice in Edinburgh,
and staff include nurses and doctors. It aims 'to
give to the patients, their families and professional attendants specialist, professional advice
and support', and to 'enable more patients to remain at home longer than might otherwise have been
possible and even die at home if that is their
wish'. The advisory service is provided by specialized nurses and the doctors in the hospice, and
only becomes involved at the request or with the
consent of the patient's general practitioner who
remains in charge of the patient. The advisory
team visits the patient, assesses his needs, and
sends written recommendations on care and management to the general practitioner. Thereafter a
nurse visits as necessary 'to monitor the drug reg-
imen, guide the family, listen and explain, inter-
pret what the doctors have said, and often to prepare them for possible admission to the hospice'.
The team often found that the usual statutory support services - including district nursing - had
not been mobilized for the patient, which suggested
lack of assessment and monitoring of the needs of
dying patients. It was felt the hospice advisory
team enabled patients to spend a longer time at
home before entering hospital or hospice care.

One study evaluating an advisory domiciliary
service based in a hospice for patients dying of
cancer is described by Parkes (1980). Spouses of
patients who had died of cancer were interviewed,
comprising: one group whose spouses had been visited by advisory team members more than once, who
were asked about the home service generally; a
group of matched pairs whose spouses had and had
not respectively received help from the home care
service; and a group of matched pairs whose spouses
had died in hospital or in the hospice respectively. It was concluded that the domiciliary service enabled patients to stay longer at home than
they did without the domiciliary service. The
costs of the domiciliary service were much less

than the cost of inpatient care to the hospice, but
the greater length of stay at home put considerable
stress upon the families and in turn therefore the
patients. However, generally the spouses felt they
had been helped by the service.

Nineteen health authorities responding to the
CNO survey reported some development in their districts to give help to the dying. These developments included the provision of Macmillan nurses
and similar schemes to give advice and expertise to
patients and community nursing staff. In some districts a district nurse advisor had been established to act as a resource person, in others a
small team undertook this work. Another type of
scheme is found in Newcastle, where two district
nursing sisters are based in a hospital pain clinic. They follow up patients who have attended the
clinic and 'also take referrals from community nurses and/or general practitioners who require help
or support in the care of terminally ill patients
in their practices'.

Support for district nurses from specialist and
liaison nurses, and from other services
From the information provided by respondents
to the CNO survey, it appeared that health authorities were establishing posts for specialist and
liaison nurses who could give support to the district nursing service in a variety of areas (other
than with the elderly or dying discussed earlier).

Specialist nurse posts had been established in
the fields of stoma care, coronary care, inconnin-
ence, orthopaedics, oncology, diabetes, mastectomy
care, mental handicap, and stroke care. Altogether
nineteen authorities reported having specialist
nurses in at least one of these fields. There was
some variation in the way these nurses were organized. In one authority, specialist nurses had been
attached to the community nursing teams, in other
authorities specialist nurses provided a service to
the nurses and patients more generally. They were
variously based in the community or the hospital,
with access to wards and out-patient clinics. The
schemes were said to be successful, and one authority reported that general practitioner and hospital
and community nursing staff had asked for the continuation and extension of the scheme providing a
stoma-care nurse specialist, and this had been
done.

Health authorities in the CNO survey reported
a number of schemes designed to help the incontin-

ent and their carers. Four authorities reported providing home laundry services for patients at home (two of these were joint funded). Four authorities had specialist incontinence nurse advisers, another one reported an advisory service and two had incontinence clinics. Advice was given to patients, relatives and nursing staff. One authority had appointed two male charge nurses to undertake changing the catheters of male genitourinary patients.

Three authorities reported schemes to help stroke patients. One authority in Lancashire had established a multidisciplinary stroke rehabilitation team, which the district nursing sister coordinated. The team comprised, apart from the district nurse, an SRN, an SEN, an occupational therapist, a physiotherapist, and a speech therapist, and aimed to improve care for stroke patients in the community. One authority had a specialised nurse to help in stroke rehabilitation, and this authority as well as one other, reported having established stroke clubs.

Nineteen health authorities in the CNO survey reported having liaison nurses in the fields of diabetics, paediatrics, maternity, chest conditions, and accident and emergency, as well as nurses to liaise generally between hospital and community. There was also a liaison nursing officer for the homeless and rootless in London (funded by inner city joint funding), and a district nurse liaising between community nursing and social services (also a joint-funded post) to provide 'home care'.

Warner (1981) in a study of hospital/community nurse liaison adds a cautionary note 'that where the liaison nurse does the liaison' (that is, is the required link between hospital and community nurses for a hospital), this is 'likely to reduce contact and therefore understanding and trust' - as well as possibly creating delay in the despatch of information. The role of the liaison nurse, however, as a facilitator of such liaison - i.e. by securing and making conveniently available the necessary up-to-date information that will help hospital and community nurses to communicate in a timely, accurate and effective fashion - is emphasized.

PRACTICE NURSES

Training courses and associations for practice nurses

Training courses designed for the needs of practice nurses and associations for them have arisen ad hoc, since no organization has been responsible for providing these needs, although it was stated in the appendix to CNO77(8) 'Nursing in Primary Health Care' that practice nurses could be included in the training programmes organized by health authorities. However, Reedy et al. (1980) in describing a survey of the characteristics of practice nurses and health authority employed nurses, found that 64% of the practice nurses had not 'received any continuing education during their present employment', compared to 29% of the health authority nurses. Also they report that 32% of practice nurses said they had access to continuing education, compared to 91% of the health authority nurses.

Courses specifically for practice nurses have been provided. Leiper (1975) describes such a course in Hampshire, and Mourin (1980) one at Norwich, both being based at further education coleges. Both reported that the nurses attending wanted further courses.

A few associations of practice nurses are mentioned - Mourin (1980) refers to a Norfolk Practice Nurses Group, formed after the course held at Norwich mentioned above, and Wrightson (1975) describes the Hull Practice Nurses Association formed back in 1972. The Royal College of Nursing has established a Practice Nurses Forum and has planned training courses (Rankin, 1981). A report by the Steering Group of the Royal College of Nursing et al. (1984) made recommendations on the training needs and curriculum for practice nurses and is summarized in Chapter Three, item 29.

The practice nurse's work in the treatment room

A number of studies have reported on the actual work undertaken by nurses - usually practice nurses - in the treatment room. Development of this type of work has been enabled not just by the employment of practice nurses who work under the direction of the general practitioner, but by the provision, particularly in health centres, of treatment rooms.

Bain and Haines (1974) reported on a survey (over 2,000 cases) of work undertaken in the treat-

ment room of a Scottish health centre. Most of the
work was done by an SEN practice nurse, who was
said to have played a valuable role in undertaking
a large volume and variety of procedures, and dealing with a large number of self-referrals from patients, about half the cases being self-referrals.
Further training for the nurse in other procedures,
and the employment of another nurse, was planned.

A study of the work in a Yorkshire health
centre treatment room provided data on over 61,000
procedures in four years (Waters et al. 1980). Most
procedures were carried out by the practice nurses
(as these procedures were not part of usual nursing
curricula) and overall 30% of procedures needed
training or initial supervision of the nurses, a
category which increased over time. The writers
argue that the extension of the nurses' work would
not have been possible if they had not been general
practitioner employees and subject instead to the
area health authority approval. Over 30% of the
patients made their initial contact with the practice nurse, who referred them if necessary to the
general practitioner.

A later study was published by the same team
(Waters and Lunn, 1981) of treatment procedures in
the same practice. Over a third of the procedures
were of the type requiring 'initial assessment or
training or both', but these were limited in variety. The practice nurses were authorized by the
doctors to undertake these procedures, but the
authors conclude that if an attached health authority nurse were to have an equal role in the treatment room, their extension of procedures would have
to be agreed with the health authority, and that
nurses should only be attached to a practice if
they were willing to train for and undertake these
procedures.

The OPCS survey (Dunnell and Dobbs, 1982)
found that general practitioner employed nurses
spent 30% of their time on technical tests and
assessments, and 47% on technical procedures, compared to 2% and 40% respectively spent on these
activities by district nurses.

Extensions of the role of the practice nurse

A study by Marriott (1981) looked at the work
of practice nurses in a group practice in Worcest-
ershire, where the patients were allowed 'open
access' to the nurse if they wished. Forty-six per
cent of patients did in fact see the nurse first,
out of a sample of 3,000 attendances. Marriott

feels that with adequate safeguards - for instance observation of the nurses' work and regular meetings between doctors and nurses to discuss problems - the doctors could confidently delegate work to nurses. Marriott feels that the care of patients is improved by this system, although he also thinks that 'further research is required to audit the management of patients by nurses when patients have open access to them'.

In one group practice in a London borough, the practice nurses undertook a new role in the running of the general practitioners' surgery sessions (Bevan et al. 1979). The nurse saw each patient in a consulting room before the doctor, took a brief history and did any preliminary examination or other preparations she felt necessary. The doctor then came in to see the patient while the nurse went on to prepare the next patient for the doctor in another consulting room. The scheme as described utilized experimental surgery premises, but was originally implemented in conventional premises at times when rooms were available to enable each doctor and nurse team to have at least two consulting rooms in operation. Doctors, nurses and patients were generally pleased with the new arrangement. In particular the system enabled the doctors to spend a higher proportion of their time 'on tasks considered central to the doctor's role', and they found their work less fatiguing.

Marsh (1976) describes how practice nurses are employed in his practice to run family planning and well-woman clinics. In family planning provision, the nurse takes over routine follow-up of patients, makes home visits if necessary and gives advice on contraception and related problems. The nurse concerned with running the well-woman clinic does relevant examinations and takes cervical smears. The system frees the doctors for other work and is an example of what the nurse, given suitable training, can undertake in a general practice setting.

Two studies describe how a nurse was involved in monitoring conditions within general practice. In one practice, a nurse (qualified also as a health visitor) employed by the practice undertook a survey of all those aged 65 years and over who were on long-term drug treatment so that they could be reviewed (Martys, 1982). The 'drug monitor' was trained by the general practitioner 'to evaluate problems associated with drug treatment and to identify drug-related morbidity occurring in elderly patients on long-term treatment'. She visited and interviewed the patient and took a blood sample. Over a third of the patients who were taking long-term drug treatment were thought to be experiencing some adverse effects and their regimens were corrected wherever possible. The 'drug monitor' nurse will be involved in regular follow-ups of patients on long-term drug treatment.

In another practice in Wales, the nurse undertook the home monitoring of blood glucose levels in diabetics (Gibbins et al. 1983). She was instructed in the self-monitoring technique by a consultant physician. Diabetic patients were seen by her and by a general practitioner to be examined and to be instructed in the blood glucose monitoring techniques, and any further management was undertaken in the practice. The authors conclude that home monitoring of blood glucose in general practice is feasible, and that if such a service is to be offered 'two essential ingredients are a well motivated practice nurse and an efficient registration and recall system for diabetic patients'.

(In the next section 'Extending the role of the nurse', an article by Martys describes a scheme in which a health visitor helped monitor adverse reactions to antibiotics.)

Not surprisingly health authorities responding to the CNO survey had little to report concerning practice nurses, who are employed by general practitioners. One authority mentioned that a practice nurse was involved in screening programmes in general practice, and another that a practice nurse had been involved in 'post basic NHS education and training on recognition and treatment of anaphylactic shock'. A third authority reported that 'practice nurses were invited to attend unit meetings of nursing officers, community oriented study days and in-service training' but that few practice nurses attended.

EXTENDING THE ROLE OF THE NURSE

'Nurse practitioners'

An increasing number of published articles are discussing the pros and cons of the concept of the 'nurse practitioner', a nurse in primary care, who could be a point of first contact for patients and could take decisions about their management - including of course the decision to refer to a doctor just as a general practitioner might refer to a specialist. It has been argued that this would be a more economic system, since nurse training is far less expensive than medical training (and nurses are paid less than doctors) and these nurses could take over part of the family doctor workload. (However, if doctors need to be at hand to supervise or deal with problems arising, the system is not necessarily more economic. See Murray, J.J. quoted in Expenditure Committee, House of Commons, 1977.) Recently the Community Nursing Review (DHSS, 1986) recommended the introduction of nurse practitioners into primary health care (see page 105).

A pilot study in Birmingham of a nurse practitioner in general practice was described by Stilwell (1981). The nurse practitioner (a qualified health visitor) held one surgery a week for six months which patients had the option of attending, or to which they had been referred by the general practitioner. The nurse practitioner referred patients to the general practitioner if this was felt to be appropriate, otherwise she gave advice about managing minor illnesses, prescribed from a limited range of drugs (the prescription being signed by the general practitioner), monitored certain conditions and gave general information about personal health care.

In a later article Stilwell (1982) describes the follow-up stage to the pilot scheme, in which the nurse practitioner provided a full-time service to patients. Consultations were kept as informal as possible, the nurse practitioner being known by her christian name. She worked with the supervision of one general practitioner in the practice with whom regular meetings were held to review tasks of both nurse practitioner and general practitioner in this system. The general practitioner suggested to patients he thought appropriate that they might see the nurse practitioner for routine follow-up consultations, an option which patients could decline. If patients saw the nurse practitioner twice about the same illness, they were requested to consult the general practitioner. The nurse practitioner used the normal medical records to record findings, she could recommend certain medications, and if these needed prescriptions, the general practitioner had to sign these (as in the pilot stage described above). Examination and treatments were based on protocols used for family nurse practitioners in the University of North Carolina, Department of Family Medicine, and agreed with the supervising general practitioner. The role of this nurse practitioner has evolved and

changed over time, for example at one stage she was
sharing the on-call rota with the general practitioner, but this was stopped on the advice of the
Medical Defence Union. Her work is to be evaluated
by the General Practice Teaching and Research Unit
at Birmingham Medical School.

In a further article on this subject, Stilwell
(1984) identifies five areas of work for the nurse
practitioner; acting as an alternative consultant
for the patient; detecting serious disease by physical examination; managing 'minor and chronic ailments and injuries'; providing health education;
and finally, counselling. She emphasizes that
nurse practitioners have their own particular role
in primary health care provision, and are not 'physician's assistants'.

The work of an SRN who for over four years was
a 'nurse practitioner' in the East End of London is
described by Cohen (1984). She held consultations
with vagrants and alcoholics, most of whom were not
registered with a general practitioner. She was
supervised by a general practitioner who prescribed
a limited range of drugs in bulk for her to dis-
pense independently. Patients were given advice on
health problems and if necessary referred to a general practitioner or a consultant. Her salary was
initially provided by a charity but was taken on in
1984 by the local health authority. However, her
surgery was closed in 1985 (Gaze 1985) when insp-
ectors from the Pharmaceutical Society confiscated
her supply of drugs, and the legality and validity
of her work has been questioned. However, the
nurse practitioner writing recently reported: 'the
DHSS however has allowed me to continue my autonomous practice' (Burke-Masters, 1986).

In contrast an experiment using a person of
quite different background and training is described by Reedy et al. (1980). A final year student
from a physician's associate programme in the USA
worked in a general practice for two months. His
work included consultations in the surgery and on
home visiting, and under supervision managed a
representative sample of cases. It is suggested
that this type of auxiliary could be useful in
under-doctored areas.

Miscellaneous 'extensions' of the nursing role
      MacGuire (1980) has argued that in the United
Kingdom 'nurses ... are quietly expanding their
roles ... to meet new demands without an accompanying fanfare of new titles'. We refer below to

some schemes and studies which illustrate possible
'extensions' of the nursing role in primary care in
the last few years. (Extensions of the role of the
practice nurse were described in the previous section above).

A clinic to treat varicose ulcers which is
'staffed and entirely run by nurses' at Staines is
described by Wilson (1977). The clinic, in a
health centre, treats patients referred by the general practitioners of the various practices in the
centre, and is staffed by the district nurses. It
is felt that the clinic saves the time of many nurses' visits, and that by being referred at an earlier stage by their general practitioners to nurses
who have expertise in ulcer treatment, better results in healing are obtained for patients.

Research nurses have been employed in general
practices as part of the MRC study of the effects
of treating hypertension (Barnes, 1981 and 1982 and
Bryan, 1982). They are trained to take blood pressures to a high degree of accuracy, take blood samples and spin them in a centrifuge to obtain serum,
to record and read ECGs and to give patients the
appropriate hypertensive drugs, all according to
the MRC protocol. In addition to their work for
the trials, it is reported that some of these nurses are undertaking further work in the practices,
setting up clinics, e.g. in hypertension for patients not in the study, or for diabetics. One
practice claims that their nurse's work has enabled
the general practitioners to increase the time they
spend on patient consultations.

Another research project is also utilizing
nurses, in trying to prevent heart disease and
strokes. Three practices in Oxfordshire are participating in a study funded by the Chest, Heart and
Stroke Association, in which nurses in general
practice give health checks to patients aged 35-64
(Anderson, 1984). The nurse checks 'blood pressure, weight, diet and smoking and drinking habits', and identifies those potentially at risk.
Then she and the general practitioner collaborate
in advising and encouraging patients to alter their
habits over a period of time. This project has
been promoted in the general practices concerned by
a 'facilitator' whose role is described by Fullard,
Fowler and Gray (1984). The facilitator (Fullard),
who is a trained health visitor and health education officer, 'helped the primary care team to set
up objectives, trained practice nurses to measure

blood pressure, and set up a system to measure the progress of the programme'.

In a small study (Whitehead, 1982) in which general practitioners and district nurses were questioned about their views of nurses undertaking hypertension clinics, response was generally favourable to the idea. The general practitioners felt it would give them more time for other patients and the SRN district nurses were keen to be involved in the prevention as well as the management of hypertension. SEN district nurses were not as enthusiastic about the idea.

Barber et al. (1976) compared in a study the decisions made by a nurse and the general practitioners of a practice about the urgency of requests for home visits. At first there was some discrepancy between the nurse and doctor assessments which potentially could put patients at risk. After actual visits and comparisons of decisions were made, it was felt that the nurse could, given suitable guidelines, assess the relative urgency of home visits and the appropriate action to take.

Marsh (1977) describes how nurses and health visitors in his practice were involved in a primary health care team effort to deal with 'minor illnesses' in his practice. The general practitioner referred follow-up of minor illness to the nurses, and patients then often took recurring episodes straight back to nurses. Nurses and health visitors gave advice about self-treatment of illness, avoiding prescriptions and encouraging patients to buy their own 'patent medicines' such as analgesics, if appropriate.

Martys (1982) describes a study in which a health visitor was involved in monitoring adverse reactions to antibiotics.

> In a general practice in Derbyshire, 298 patients who had been given antibiotics were questioned about possible adverse reactions to the drug prescribed. Four methods of assessing adverse effects of drugs in the community were used, and a comparison was made of the replies elicited from patients by doctor and health visitor respectively. Significant differences were shown to occur in the way in which each investigator completed the questionnaires. If ancillary staff are to be employed in monitoring adverse effects of drugs in the community on a large scale then they will have to use a method less reliant on

the differentiation of incidental symptoms
from drug side effects than is required in the
present survey.

Martys considers that:

to obtain information on a large scale about
adverse effects of drugs in the community the
help of paramedical or ancillary staff workers
would be essential.

A research health visitor has described her
role in a research project, funded by the community
nursing service in Paddington and North Kensington
Health Authority (Drennan, 1985 and Drennan (undated ?1985)). The project, which lasted 18 months,
began in 1983 and was done 'to examine how health
visitors can work within existing community groups
to promote awareness of health and the health services'. The health visitor had no family caseload,
aiming to work with groups of people rather than
with individuals as is usual in health visiting.
As she writes:

I went to community organisations, associations and groups and offered my services as a
health visitor. I gave information, initiated
discussions, organised health courses and sessions and provided a catalyst to look at
health issues.

The techniques used to evaluate the project comprised 'a detailed field diary', analysis of 'the
client's perspectives by canvassing "key" people
such as group leaders and community workers to obtain comments' and examination of the agendas of
the groups the health visitor had worked with.
Evaluation showed that the health visitor had had
some effect on both local health services and community organisations. It was also reported that
'this project has shown that there is an unmet need
for groups of people to have access to a health
professional to talk about health in a positive,
holistic sense, in familiar settings'.

Attitudes towards extending the nurse's role
Some surveys have been done of patients' and
doctors' views on extending the nurse's role, and
three are mentioned here. A few practices already
use nurses to make home visits, but in one practice
where this is done, a patient survey found that 41%

of patients would not like the nurse to appear if
they had requested a home visit from the doctor.
Patients who had received home visits from the
nurse were generally satisfied with their treatment
although a quarter would still have preferred to
see the doctor (Marsh and Kaim Caudle, 1976).
    Bowling (1981,a,b,c) reports on a sample sur-
vey of doctors' and nurses' attitudes towards delegation of tasks to nurses. Less than half the general practitioners regularly delegated minor clinical procedures. They were generally against the
nurse being the first contact for the patient in
the survey although they were more prepared to send
the nurse on a home visit to assess if the patient
needed to see the doctor. More nurses than doctors
were in favour of nurses doing these 'decision-
making' tasks such as seeing the patient for initial screening.
    Miller and Backett (1980) in a larger survey
of general practitioner opinions, found that 45% of
general practitioners would permanently accept having a family practice nurse 'who would undertake
after suitable training, tasks including history
taking, examination, diagnosis and advice on treatment'. Nearly a third were against having such a
person in the practice, the rest had no strong view
or would accept such a person temporarily where
there was a shortage of general practitioners.
    A number of surveys of patients' opinions and
experiences relating to the nurse's role were carried out in the practice in which one extension of
the practice nurse's role was evaluated (see page
165). Bevan et al. (1979) concluded:

> It appears that the respondents were generally
> favourable to the nurse in her supportive role
> as a caring or motherly figure and to her
> undertaking minor clinical procedures. They
> were more reluctant to accept the nurse in a
> decision-making role, at least without some
> assurance either by direct experience or by
> information from their doctors that any
> developments of this kind were appropriate.

From these surveys it appears that nurse
practitioners would have a mixed reception from
general practitioners, nurses and patients, but a
considerable number of all groups would support
such an innovation.
    Another survey carried out by Bowling (1985)
was concerned with the policies of district health

authorities towards extending the clinical role of
the nurse in general practice. Of the 192 districts in England surveyed, 64% listed clearly what
tasks could be delegated to nurses. It was reported that:

> Although 71% of the DNSs [Directors of Nursing
> Services] questioned said a policy on the ex-
> tended role of the nurse had been drawn up in
> their districts, few met all three criteria
> recommended by the DHSS: specific task def-
> inition, training requirements and legal safe-
> guards.

The author concludes:

> If all the districts issued uniform, detailed
> guidelines, the confusion over "the extended
> role" might be further reduced... For this to
> be satisfactorily achieved, it is essential
> for the DHSS to give guidance and support.

Two developments in the role of the nurse, already referred to in the discussion of the literature above, were mentioned by health authorities
responding to the CNO survey, namely the introduction of a nurse practitioner in Birmingham, and
the involvement of district nurses in varicose
ulcer clinics.

Two authorities responding to the CNO survey
reported schemes in which district nurses helped in
coronary care. In a research project in Notting-
ham, specially trained district nurses visited patients' homes to take ECGs and blood samples (for
cardiac enzymes) and liaised with the coronary care
unit. In Whitstable, Kent, district nurses fitted
recorders to cardiac patients for 24-hour monitoring, the recording being analysed at the district
general hospital.

GENERAL REVIEW OF SCHEMES AND STUDIES

Several publications have brought together
information on numbers of schemes and studies,
including ones in the field of community nursing,
and these are referred to below.

Three of these are concerned with schemes for
the elderly. In 'A Sourcebook of Initiatives in
the Community Care of the Elderly' (Ferlie, 1982)
over 200 schemes in England in this area are described, most in some detail. Information for the

sourcebook was obtained by approaching social service departments, health authorities, housing departments and voluntary organizations, and many of
the schemes described are concerned with domiciliary care of the elderly. Clarke (1984) looks at
the development of 'domiciliary services for the
elderly', as well as current developments and possible future trends. The book includes ample references, as does another book concerned with 'innovations in the care of the elderly' by Isaacs and
Evers (1984) which 'took place in and around Birmingham in the late 1970s and early 1980s'.
   'Primary Care Nursing' edited by Lisbeth
Hockey (1983) includes chapters on health visiting
and district nursing in the United Kingdom which
give concise summaries of developments in these
fields, with full lists of references.
   A list of briefly described schemes in community nursing is included in a report on information obtained from chief nursing officers in England (Baker and Bevan, 1983).
   A summary and discussion of 37 studies of the
work of the health visitor in the period 1960-80 in
the United Kingdom has been written by Clark
(1981). The studies include both published and
unpublished research involving data collection.
   Schemes to set up local support groups for
parents and families in which health visitors have
been involved are listed in an article by De'Ath
(1982). References and addresses for information
are given.
   A book describing innovations in the field of
preventive health care in pregnancy and early
childhood (Dowling, 1983) includes schemes involving health visitors and district nurses. The
information was obtained by approaching AHAs, CHCs
and voluntary organizations, and inviting responses
in journals; references to the individuals who gave
information, as well as to the literature are
included.

IDEAS FOR FUTURE DEVELOPMENTS

   Ideas for future developments in community
nursing which we found in the literature, or which
were given by respondents to the chief nursing
officer survey, are summarized below. Some of
these ideas are similar to developments which have
already taken place, and it is possible that some
ideas have already been put into practice, unknown
to us.

Developments in the last decade

Community nursing generally

Changes in the organization of community nursing have been suggested. Kratz (1983), looking for more autonomy for community nursing staff, puts forward the idea of 'a self-employed nursing service, on terms similar to those pertaining to the other services regulated by FPCs'. An editorial in the Journal of the Royal College of General Practitioners (1983), considering primary health care teams, speculates:

> Perhaps we will see the introduction of partnerships for some nurses. If nurses are treated as part of a practice rather than an appendage, they might then feel a greater commitment to its aims.

Baker and Bevan (1983) argued that attachment had organizational complications for a nursing officer's relationship with subordinate community nurses and general practitioners to whom they were attached.

> It may indeed be that the nursing officer's role in relation to attached community nurses is not appropriately that of a line-manager. Arguably the act of attachment to general practice implies one of detachment of the nurses in question from the Health Authority, and the nursing officer for the duration of the attachment exercises only the residual role of adviser and arbitrator on request, and constitutes a channel of information on DHSS and Health Authority policy and developments. Thus it may be that one would be thinking of an "attachment agreement" as between the health authority on the one hand and practice(s) making up a group of family doctors on the other for a defined period of years in which each party, as it were nursing and general medical, agrees to operate within broad lines essentially set down by the respective professions rather than the Health Authority. This approach might be a means of assimilating suitably qualified practice nurses into the team - as a nursing "partner" in the group practice of nurses.
> Also particularly if we are thinking of teams of the larger kind described above - 'group practices' of nurses attached to group practices of doctors - there may be a need for

a nurse equivalent to the senior partner for the team of nurses. Such a senior nursing partner would be more suitably "first-among-equals" than the line manager if her role was to parallel that of the senior general practitioner partner, given the variety of specialised disciplines to be found within the group of nurses in question. (A nurse with a role with some affinities to this was the nurse co-ordinator referred to in Gilmore et al. 1974).

A central feature of the Community Nursing Review Teams's recommendations (DHSS, 1986) was, as we have seen (see page 101), the formation of neighbourhood nursing teams each managed by a neighbourhood nursing manager based in the neighbourhood. The review team also proposed that as one means of promoting primary health care team work,

> to establish and be recognised as a primary health care team, each general medical practice and the community nurses associated with it should come to an understanding of the team's objectives and individuals' roles within it.
> That understanding should be incorporated into a written agreement signed jointly by the practice partners and by the manager of the neighbourhood nursing services on behalf of the relevant health authority...

Some writers have suggested combining roles in community nursing. Keywood (1978) wanted to see a trial scheme of a triple duty nurse, combining the roles of health visiting, district nursing and midwifery, and Hicks (1976) argued that there was a case for combining the roles of district nurse and health visitor. (In some remote areas, for instance Scottish islands, nurses do already combine roles to provide a service.) Russell (1975) has advocated having 'a general nursing practitioner', a nurse specially trained from the outset for work in the community, most of the training being done in the community and not in hospital. She would combine the roles of midwife, district nurse and health visitor, and undertake follow-up visits for the general practitioner, assess needs, immunize, carry out routine maternity care and make regular visits to the elderly and the chronic sick.
A recommendation that occupational health nurses should be members of the primary health care

team is made by Slaney (1984). They would be based at health centres, have a caseload of local working units (such as shops, banks, industries etc.) and help with health education and the prevention of occupational accidents.

One respondent to the CNO survey suggested that community nursing staff should have two-way radio telephones.

Health Visiting

As mentioned above, some suggestions have been made that health visiting roles could be combined with district nursing, and possibly midwifery. Dingwall (1977) thought that in remote rural areas, the roles of health visiting and social worker could be combined. In addition he argues that it could be desirable for some health visitors to have a non-nursing background, as more training in social science is needed for the health visiting role.

The Court Report (DHSS, 1976) proposed that there should be 'child health visitors' specializing in the preventive and curative care of children under 16, and assisted by child health nurses. One suggestion from the CNO survey was that hospital paediatric nurses should undertake follow-up of patients in the community in liaison with health visitors. Mothers who were interviewed in a survey of consumer opinion about health visiting services wanted their health visitors to be mothers themselves (Field et al. 1982). The authors suggest that married health visitors with children could be given preference in recruitment to health visiting, and part-time work made available to health visitors as an alternative to their giving up entirely to bring up their children.

Finally, one respondent to the CNO survey suggested that health visitors could work in teams.

District nursing

Fry (1984) would like to see the ratio of doctors to nurses in the community re-examined. 'Rather than having two general practitioners to one SRN, the ratio should be reversed' he writes, so that nurses can give more help to those caring for the sick and elderly at home. One respondent to the CNO survey suggested that extra district nursing staff could be funded from the money allocated to FPCs to fund practice nurses. The Community Nursing Review Report (DHSS, 1986) also made a recommendation of this kind (see page 105). Two respondents to the CNO survey wanted district nurses to have access to hospital beds for terminal care and short-term relief cases. (One scheme which nearly provides this is found in Burford Community Hospital - see section on intensive home nursing, page 153.)

Two suggestions from the CNO survey related specifically to the care of the elderly. One was that district nurses should be joint funded, to service residential homes for the elderly; the other was that nurses (or auxiliary visitors) should work as one unit with the elderly

> so that the role demarcation is not clearly defined, and the role of regular visitor, who is known to the old person, can alter with any increased nursing need.

An additional role for the district nurse is envisaged by Anderson (1983) who thinks that she could have 'a key role to play in the provision of care to patients on CAPD home dialysis treatment', with the current emphasis on care in the home rather than in the hospital.

A radical scheme proposed by one respondent to the CNO survey was that, experimentally, there could be

> rotation of community staff between community and hospital, to assess effectiveness in providing continuity of care, practicability and cost effectiveness.

One nurse (at the time Divisional Nursing Officer, Community) suggested that older district nurses who were experienced but perhaps unable to do the heavy work that nursing patients at home could demand, should be employed as treatment room nurses, jointly financed by the health authority and the FPC (Gray, 1982).

There were ideas concerned with the provision of care assistants who combined the roles of a 'home help' type person with more personal care of patients. One respondent to the CNO survey wanted these staff to be employed by the NHS. (At present these staff seem to be mainly employed by social service departments, although in at least one authority they are joint funded, and of course nursing auxiliaries carry out part of the care assistant type role. In addition there are schemes involving volunteers.) Two writers had similar views on the development of these care assistants. Muir Gray

179

Developments in the last decade

(1977) suggested that a 'primary care worker' be developed 'with common training for those staff who are at present labelled home helps, care assistants, nursing auxiliaries, wardens of sheltered housing, and occupational therapy and physiotherapy aides'. Hopkins (1984) proposed one-year training for 'a new type of caring and rehabilitation worker in the essential aspects of practical help' for elderly and disabled people. They would replace the care at present provided by a multiplicity of staff.

Extending the role of the nurse
    A proposal that district nurses could take on 'a monitoring and counselling role' is made by Faulkner (1983), so that they would be involved in the psychological as well as the physical needs of patients, giving 'total patient care'. One respondent to the CNO survey suggested there could be a nurse adviser at the surgery, for health promotion, non-medical problems, and counselling. As Kratz (1982) has argued, in order for nurses to expand their sphere of expertise, they need to identify new approaches to nursing tasks and 'new tasks or target populations for themselves'.
    In a number of articles, Saint-Yves has advocated his scheme for a new system of primary health care summed up in Saint-Yves, (1983) in which the general practitioner is no longer the first point of contact for the patient, but is instead 'a specialist generalist' providing a 24-hour back-up service. Three new categories of paramedical staff would be specially trained, namely the clinical associate, the community nurse, and the nursing aide. The first of these is the most senior, and the point of first contact. The clinical associate

> would provide an initial emergency service, make a first diagnosis, treat the commonly occurring illnesses, prescribe from a restricted list of drugs and run routine clinics such as surgeries, ante and post-natal, immunisation and contraceptive clinics.

    A proposal for a common basic training in medicine and nursing is made by Chant (1982). This training would produce a 'stem doctor' who could then go on to specialize as a doctor or nurse, or as an administrator in the health service, utilizing the variety of post-graduate courses at present on offer.

Chapter Five

EVALUATIVE RESEARCH ON DEVELOPMENTS IN COMMUNITY
NURSING PUBLISHED FROM 1974 TO THE PRESENT

INTRODUCTION

In the last chapter we considered developments
implemented in community nursing since 1974 as well
as untried ideas proposed in the literature or
elsewhere. In this chapter we concentrate only on
the published reports mentioned in Chapter Four in
which there was, in our judgement, some attempt
made at a rational evaluation of the development as
implemented - that is, where an attempt was made to
collect and discuss factual evidence on the working
out in practice of the development. In a chart -
see pages 204-9 - we have classified each of these
studies according to a number of characteristics
relevant in our opinion to the quality of the evidence in relation to an evaluation of the development. (In Baker et al. (1984) most of these studies are summarized in greater detail than is here
possible.) In the next section we define these
characteristics and explain their relevance. In
the final section of this chapter, we review the
whole body of these studies, which constitutes as
far as we have been able to discover, the bulk of
the completed and disseminated research project
activity which comes within our terms of reference.

There are two broad questions to be asked of
an evaluative study:
1.   Can we rely on the evidence presented on which
     the conclusions are based?
2.   If so, how useful is the evidence in answering
     the kinds of practical questions which those
     who are considering whether or not to imple-
     ment the development ought to ask in order to
     come to an informed decision?
There are a number of facets of a study which throw
some light on these matters, some are no more than

181

common sense, others are concerned with more technical aspects of research methods.

CHARACTERISTICS OF REPORTS ON EVALUATIONS OF
DEVELOPMENTS AND AN EXPLANATION OF TERMS AND
ABBREVIATIONS USED IN THE CHART ON PAGES 204-9

The sub-headings in this section are those of
the columns of the chart (see pages 204-9). In the
corresponding sub-sections we first explain the
sub-heading and any abbreviations or terms used in
the corresponding column of the chart, and then
briefly where appropriate discuss and justify the
inclusion of the characteristic.

Study identifier
The studies are: classified and arranged by
subject in the same way as in Chapter Four; identified by the number corresponding to that subject
(before the 'decimal point') and, after the 'decimal point', by the number of the study within the
subject category. The studies are arranged in al-
phabetical order of (first named) author and,
within a given subject and for a given author, by
year of publication. The studies referred to in
the chart are listed in the references to Chapter
Four where they are distinguished by the study identifier used in the chart.

Year
This is the year of publication. (In a few
cases more than one year is given since our information on the research is based on more than one
publication.) Year of publication of a report is
almost invariably available and at least indicates
the minimum age of the information provided (though
this may have been gathered some time before publication). How far the passage of time has rendered
findings obsolete depends on the nature of the
innovation reported and significant intervening
events. In fact during the period with which this
book is concerned, in many spheres of community
nursing, little happened to render out-of-date a
good study say on the impact of attachment or of
the work of a specialist-type of community nurse -
though of course what were novelties in 1975 may be
relatively commonplace today. However, changes in
organization and management arrangements for community nurses might render the conclusions of studies on the impact of superseded management patterns
irrelevant.

Journal or publisher

This is the name of the journal, or publisher of the book or booklet. Where the findings of the study were reported in two or more publications, a separate line is used for each one in the chart. The following abbreviations are used for journals or publishers:

AA	Age and Ageing
BJS	British Journal of Surgery
BMJ	British Medical Journal
CCHD	Child Care and Health Development
CETHV	Council for the Education and Training of Health Visitors
CH	Croom Helm
HB	Health Bulletin
HSSJ	Health and Social Service Journal
HV	Health Visitor
JCN	Journal of Community Nursing
JDN	Journal of District Nursing (Formerly Journal of Community Nursing)
JECH	Journal of Epidemiology and Community Health
JPS	Journal of Pediatric Surgery
JRCGP	Journal of the Royal College of General Practitioners
JRSS	Journal of the Royal Statistical Society
LA	The Lancet
MHVCN	Midwife, Health Visitor and Community Nurse
NM	Nursing Mirror
NPHT	Nuffield Provincial Hospitals Trust (strictly speaking the Oxford University Press publishes for NPHT)
NT	Nursing Times (NM and NT now combined)
PRACT	The Practitioner
PGMJ	Postgraduate Medical Journal
PH	Public Health
RCN	Royal College of Nursing
RR	Research Report (i.e. not published in usual sense)

The journal and sometimes publisher of a book, where this is published for say a professional body, can in subtle ways affect the emphasis of a report. For example a paper on a particular nursing development in a medical journal may differ from a report on the same development in a nursing

journal in its description of, and attitude towards, the roles say of medically qualified and
nurse participants (we don't say it will - but the
critical reader should at least have the question
in mind in reading the paper).

Author type(s)
    These are the various types of author of the
publications. Where a publication has several
authors of the same type, that type will of course
only be listed once in the chart, where the following abbreviations are used:

Anon	No authors' names given in public-ation
Chem	Member of British Pharmaceutical Society
Psych	Clinical psychologist
D	Medical practitioner (further information not available)
DN	Person with district nursing qual-ifications (excluding those listed under NO, see below) and/or pract-ising as a district nurse
GP	General medical practitioner
HD	Hospital doctor (of any kind includ-ing consultants)
HV	Health visitor (excluding those des-cribed as NO, see below, but includ-ing anyone with health visitor qualifications even though not nec-essarily practising as a health visitor)
N	Person with nursing qualifications (but no other information given in publication)
NO	Person with nursing qualifications (including possibly health visiting and/or district nursing qualifica-tions) listed as being of the rank of nursing officer or above within the NHS
NS	Type of author not stated
PN	Practice nurse
RW	Research worker, with neither nur-sing nor medical qualifications
SCM	Specialist in community medicine
SS	Person working from local authority social services department

Note - where an * is placed against an author type, e.g. NO*, GP*, this means at least one of the authors of the type indicated is described as having a specific research function e.g.NO (research). This is not done in the case of SCM or RW, since they are by definition deemed to have a research and intelligence function.

The background of the author(s) may affect the conclusions of the paper. For example it is easy to see differences of view as between medically qualified writers and those with nursing qualifications in discussing the nursing process. A multidisciplinary team of authors relating to a paper concerning the disciplines in question is one safeguard against disciplinary bias - or indeed individual prejudices - but even here a dominant personality may affect conclusions. The presence among the authors of some reputable lay-research worker may help to hold the ring amongst differing professionals' entrenched views. (Discerning readers may detect a bias on the part of the authors of this book in this last statement!)

Location(s) of study

For studies within England the Regional Health Authority is given (abbreviations given below) and in the case of the four Thames regions, we have indicated whether or not the location was in the 'Greater London Area'. For studies outside England we have indicated only the country, viz. Scotland, Wales or Northern Ireland. (We confined our search to studies in the United Kingdom. We have also indicated whether the study was undertaken in an urban (u), rural (r) or mixed (m) area (except where the area is indicated as being within the 'Greater London Area').

The abbreviations used are as follows

SET	South East Thames Regional Health Authority area
NET	North East Thames Regional Health Authority area
SWT	South West Thames Regional Health Authority area
NWT	North West Thames Regional Health Authority area

(The use of L in addition to the above indicates that the location was in the 'Greater London Area'.)

EA	East Anglia Regional Health Authority area
MERSEY	Mersey Regional Health Authority area
N	Northern Regional Health Authority area
NW	North Western Regional Health Authority area
OX	Oxford Regional Health Authority area
SW	South Western Regional Health Authority area
TRENT	Trent Regional Health Authority area
WM	West Midlands Regional Health Authority area
WESS	Wessex Regional Health Authority area
YORKS	Yorkshire Regional Health Authority area
Various	Several locations in England and Scotland. Not precisely described.
NI	Northern Ireland
SCOT	Scotland
W	Wales

In principle there is a lot one would like to know about the location(s) in which a development was tried out. For someone contemplating introducing a development, the fact that it was successful in a similar area to his or hers is obviously one point to be borne in mind - as are particular opportunities or difficulties associated with areas where the development was studied. To the extent that the development was successful in a variety of locations, one's confidence that it is likely to be generally so is strengthened - this matter is taken up in the section headed 'scale'.

A pilot or preliminary study (or interim report)?
That is, is the study one which is described as a preliminary to a fuller study, or the report as an interim one on the study with the implication that something more substantial is to follow? (These do not always materialize as, for example, sometimes the findings of the pilot suggest there is no point in proceeding to a full study.)
Abbreviations used:

Y	Yes
N	No
Y?	Probably a pilot or preliminary study

Self-evidentally, conclusions from a pilot study or those otherwise of an interim nature are usually based on more limited evidence than it is envisaged would emerge from the full study and have to be treated as tentative. However, research workers sometimes receive research support for a pilot study with support for the full study being conditional on the outcome of the pilot (both in terms of the success of the development and the quality of the research effort). This sometimes means that the quality of the research at the pilot stage is high, simply because so much depends on it. Again this consideration does put pressure on the research workers or innovators not to lightly dismiss a development particularly if their future livelihood depends on a full study going ahead. We are not suggesting that results are consciously or even necessarily at all affected by such considerations - but it as well to be aware of the pressures that exist.

Controlled trial?

A controlled trial is one in which the development under study is tried out on a group of individuals or other basic and indivisible units (some times called experimental units) for the purpose of the trial (e.g. 'households' or 'mother and baby'): the results are compared with those of the conventional and/or possibly other alternatives to the development, also tried out on a group of experimental units (the control group) in such a way as to make the comparison of the development and conventional alternative(s) as fair as possible. The classical model of a controlled trial is the clinical trial where a new drug is tried out on a group of patients and the conventional one (or possibly an inert preparation, i.e. a placebo) on another 'control' group - in such a way as to make comparison between the two regimens as fair as possible. Of course, the fairness of the trial is helped by making the two groups of subjects, those receiving the development and the controls respectively, as alike as possible. Indeed one design for a trial, the 'paired comparison', does essentially involve finding pairs of subjects as alike as possible with respect to characteristics thought likely to be relevant to the comparison, and giving one of each pair the development regime and the other the conventional or placebo. Indeed sometimes it is possible to use a subject as his/her own control by giving the subject for one period of the study the developmental regime and for the other the conventional regime. In this last case a further refinement in design is the 'crossover trial'. Here each experimental unit receives first one treatment then the other, but because the order in which an individual receives the treatment may affect the response observed, experimental units are randomly assigned to two groups - in one of which the development is applied first, then the control; in the case of the second, the control treatment is applied first and then the development.

The design of trials, so as to make them as fair as possible in the comparisons made between treatment and the consideration, is a large subject and the interested reader is referred for details to books such as Hill (1984) and Cox (1958). In this section we are simply interested in whether the study contained a control group of any kind. Some studies just provide details of the development as tried out and compare the results, if at all, with say the situation before the development was introduced. The essence of a controlled trial is that the research workers have some control over the composition of the experimental and control groups respectively (and the environment in which they are tested).

In contrast to a controlled trial, a survey is simply the study of a number of units chosen from a population of interest so as to make them as representative as convenient of that population. The purpose of a survey may be simply to estimate some characteristic of the population - for example, in a survey of the population of children aged 10 to 14 inclusive in a certain area, to estimate the proportion who smoke more than five cigarettes per week or perhaps the average number of cigarettes smoked per child in that population per week - or it may be to look for associations between characteristics of interest - e.g. do relatively heavy smokers tend to have more or less accidents on average than non-smokers? Note that in the case of a survey designed to explore associations, there is no attempt at control of the 'treatment-like' characteristic under study - here level of smoking. Accordingly any association does not necessarily imply a causal link. Even if heavy smokers do tend to have more accidents than non-smokers, it would be going beyond the evidence of the survey to assert that smoking tended <u>to lead</u> to accidents - that might be so, but it could be that having accidents leads to smoking or that some other

unexplained characteristic tends to cause people both to have accidents and to smoke heavily.
Abbreviations used:

Y   Yes

N   No

NA   Not applicable - e.g. where the emphasis was on whether the development was feasible, or where the purpose of the inquiry was to assess the effects of screening.

MM   Denotes use of a mathematical model to compare the control and experimental situations experimentally. Here the controlled trial is not performed on real subjects but on a logical (and in its behaviour, as realistic as possible) model of the real world constructed and investigated 'within' a computer (rather as tests of aspects of the development of a new aeroplane are carried out in a wind tunnel rather than using a real aeroplane). Such studies are sometimes called simulation studies.

Random selection or allocation?

Almost inevitably any development is tried out on a sub-group or sample of the total 'population' (using this word in its technical sense as the totality of people or other units under consideration) to which it is at the time of the study applicable, and the same remarks apply of course in the case of a controlled trial, to the alternative(s) with which the development is compared. So the questions to be asked are: how are the units which are to be exposed to the development and the alternative(s) respectively to be selected, and, how is it to be decided as to which 'treatment' (the development or an alternative) any particular individual shall receive?

The ideal is that the sample receiving any particular treatment shall be representative of the population as a whole to which the treatment is applicable and, in the case of a controlled trial, that the comparison between the development and alternatives shall be fair.

The goal of representativeness implies that the sample shall have similar (or at least specified) proportions of members in various categories thought important, e.g. age/sex and/or social class, but that the actual decision as to whether any individual is or is not included in the sample, is left to a chance process - so that consciously or unconsciously no kind of selective bias is allowed to creep in. For example, if one is sampling from an age/sex register of a particular practice list and wanting a sample with specified proportions of members in various age/sex groups, it would be a matter of, in principle, putting the names of all the practice population in any particular age/sex group of interest, e.g. women aged 65 to 74 years inclusive, into a hat, shaking well and drawing the required number of names from the hat as in a lottery. (In practice one does not have to actually go through this process but the principle is either the same or a convenient variant called systematic random sampling. In this latter case, if say one wants a one in ten sample from the group in question, then one chooses randomly a number between one and ten, say this turns out to be six, and takes 'systematically' every tenth name in the list, starting with the sixth, i.e. the sixth, sixteenth, twenty-sixth ... and so on.)

Sometimes a population is not divided into sub-groups for sampling purposes and the entire composition is left to chance without therefore any attempt at all on the part of the researchers to control the proportions in any sub-group.

In the case of the decision in a controlled trial as to which individual should be exposed to the development and which to the alternative(s), this should be left to chance to avoid any question of bias being introduced by either the researcher or persons in charge of the cases in the trial. (If for ethical reasons the person in charge of the management of a patient feels that for that individual patient, the decision cannot be left to chance, that individual should be excluded from the trial and given the appropriate treatment.) For example, in the case of a paired comparison trial design, where pairs of individuals are selected, as alike as possible with regard to factors thought important, and one exposed to the development and the other to the alternative, the matter of which individual should be exposed to which treatment should be decided by a chance mechanism, e.g. by tossing a coin in the case of each pair.

The abbreviations used in this column in the chart on pages 204-9 are:

Y	Yes, random selection/allocation used (see preceding column for whether or not the study took the form of a controlled trial)
TE	No, random selection/allocation method was not used and the study 'sample' included the total number of persons falling into some defined category (e.g. all those seen for the first time at a particular clinic during a particular calendar year)
N	No, random selection/allocation method not used and the sample selected by some other method than TE mentioned above.

Note: sometimes a study was made up of several parts where selection or allocation procedures varied. Where this happened more than one of the above abbreviations will be used, e.g. Y/TE.

Scale

Two matters are considered under this heading.

The first is concerned with the number of units (i.e. clients, patients or similar) on which the study is based. Where the study consisted of more than one sub-study, the number of units studied respectively in the smallest/largest sub-studies are given. Note: in the case of a survey, the number given is the number approached, not respondents, which will be fewer. Generally figures have been rounded down to the nearest ten or hundred, depending on the number of units involved.

The second matter is concerned with the number and type of sites or geographical areas in which the development was introduced and investigated.

Typically an entry in this column of the chart is a number followed by a site type or geographical area: e.g. 2 HD means the study took place over two health districts. The following abbreviations are used for site types/geographical areas:

GP	General (medical) practice
CL	Clinic
PHCT	Primary health care team
HC	Health centre
H	Hospital
DGH	District general hospital
HD	Health district

LAD	Local authority district
LB	London borough
NA	Not applicable, where the number of units studied are so few as to make irrelevant the population from which they were sampled.

Sometimes different parts of the study relate to different sites or areas, e.g. 2 GP/LAD (i.e. the study relates in part to two general practices and in part covers a local authority district).

Sometimes a study relates to only part of the indicated geographical area, e.g. part LAD or one sector of HD.

Both these matters (see page 191) are concerned with the extent to which the conclusions of a study can be generalized. Clearly results relating to a development tried out on only a few clients inspire less confidence, other things being equal, than those from a study where a much larger group of clients were involved in the investigation.

As mentioned earlier, however, sheer numbers are not the only consideration - the way the units to be studied are chosen and treatments (the development or alternative(s)) are allocated to units is also at least as important. In particular the representativeness of the samples on which the rival treatments are tried out with respect to the population of units about which it is wished to draw conclusions is very important.

Again other things being equal, the larger the number of sites (particularly if also varied in character) at which the development, and any alternatives, are tried out, the easier it will be for the reader to judge whether the conclusions drawn are likely to apply to her/his particular situation

One problem with one-site studies is that this is not infrequently a location where the person who thought up the development works and that person may well be one of the originators of the report. If so he/she may well be consciously or unconsciously convinced of the value of the development and find it difficult to deal dispassionately with the evidence collected if this runs counter to this belief. Often of course the originator of the development bends over backwards to be fair in her/his appraisal - but it is very useful to have the development tried out at a second site where those involved in implementing it are not those who thought it up in the first place.

Information included on:

Input This is information on resources needed to introduce and maintain the development in question.

S   means - yes, information provided on staff resources needed
C   means - yes, information provided on cash needed
(Often information on both types of input are provided.)
*   - denotes information given on costs of <u>study</u> as distinct from implementation of development
In one case, it was asserted that 'no resources would be required' and this was indicated by 'none required'.

The importance of indicating the resources needed to implement and run the development, as compared with those required in the case of alternatives is obvious since any comparison of other advantages and disadvantages of the various regimes is of limited use without a knowledge of the associated costs.

Outcome. This is information on the consequences for clients (and/or sometimes other interested parties) of the implementation of the development as compared with those of alternatives. In some cases it is more appropriate to think of outcome in terms of the consequences for certain parts of the health services, if the purpose of the development is to say ease pressure on those parts and to hold the quality of care for clients at a fixed level.

Clearly, knowledge of the outcomes associated with various alternative policies or practices is extremely important to decision makers when choosing which to implement or recommend.

Abbreviations used:

Y   Information based substantially on quantitive (and relatively objective) study (i.e. not mainly subjective)
Su   Information based on subjective assessment
YSu   Information based substantially on subjective assessment but with some resort to more objective data

Evaluative research on developments

> Co   Survey of consumer opinion on development
> undertaken
> NA   Not applicable

Note: Outcome is not to be confused with the output of a development and the alternatives with which it is compared. Output is essentially concerned with the level and characteristics of activities associated with the development or other alternative regimes - and information about this is almost invariably given in reports of studies. What output does not say anything about are the consequences of these activities for clients or other interested parties.

AN ANALYSIS OF THE CHARACTERISTICS OF STUDIES AND PUBLICATIONS INCLUDED IN THE CHART ON PAGES 204-9

Subjects of studies

Of the 77 studies we considered, 48 related to the work of health visitors, 29 to that of district nurses and eight to that of practice nurses (a few studies related to the work of more than one category of nurse).

Screening and surveillance of various age groups was the subject of 24 studies, 16 of these were concerned with the elderly; with the remainder evenly divided between other adults and the very young. Predictably, health visitors were the staff mostly concerned with screening and surveillance but district nurses were involved in six of the 24 studies (mostly those concerned with the elderly) (see Table 1). A number of other studies (mainly those in which the health visitor was the type of worker primarily involved) also related to anticipatory care. In particular this is the case for most of those concerned with 'health visitors and family and child health' and 'liaison and intervention schemes for the elderly' (those in which health visitors were involved) - in the sense of finding out what people want and/or need and offering advice in the light of this information).

Under the three headings 'health visitors liaising between hospital and community services', 'health visitors and psycho-social problems' and 'specialization in health visiting', are included a total of 11 studies of health visitors in specialized and/or unconventional roles. Thus studies have been made of health visitors assisting clients (children and adults) with psycho-social problems both on an individual basis and in groups, and liaising between paediatric, maternity, accident and emergency, rehabilitation and oncology hospital departments and health and other services in the community - including one study of a child health visitor akin to that suggested by the Court Report (DHSS et al. 1976). i.e. where her work included supervising the home nursing of ill children. There have been studies too of health visitors developing specialized skills in the care of children with Down's syndrome and in the use of the Portage approach to helping developmentally delayed young children and their families. However it is clear from the references to Chapter Four, that only a small proportion of the developments of this kind have been studied at all systematically, even among those reported in the literature or otherwise brought to our notice.

Four studies were concerned with the provision of health visitor services out-of-normal working hours - arguably a response partly to the changing life styles of one of their main client groups, mothers of young children, and partly in order to reduce the need for emergency calls on general practitioner and other acute services.

Only two studies were concerned with the provision of district nursing services out-of-normal working hours. However, eight other studies were found (classified under the headings of 'intensive home nursing', 'liaison and intervention schemes for the elderly' and 'nursing and related care - joint schemes with social services') which were concerned with the provision of nursing and other care necessary for keeping relatively sick or frail people in their own homes or similar accommodation rather than in institutions, such as hospitals. Three of these studies (classified under 'nursing and related care - joint schemes with social services') related to the use of care assistants, with no formal nursing or social work qualifications, providing augmented general and domestic help necessary to keep patients in the community. In addition, two studies were concerned with the district nurse's role in day surgery and early discharge, and there were two studies relating to paediatric home nursing, one function of this specialized service being to ensure that children were able to return to their homes as quickly as possible after hospital care. Finally, there were three studies on support services for community nurses in the care of the dying which also arguably represented an exploration of a means of maintaining another category of patients in the community. Thus in all some 17 studies were concerned with the problems faced by district nurses (and some of their solutions) resulting from the policy to shift health care as far as possible from hospitals to the community - though this is a very large field in terms of the variety of medical conditions, range of circumstances and characteristics of patients and of the local health services themselves.

We only identified one study concerned with hospital-community liaison relating to district nurses as providing the liaison. Several studies were identified in which at least one feature of the developments under investigation was a district nurse or health visitor liaising between the health services and the social services.)

Seven studies related to organizational aspects of community nursing, mostly concerning the issues of attachment versus geographical allocation of staff. One did, amongst other things, look at the organization and administration of nurses within primary health care teams and two were concerned with aspects of clerical help for health visitors.

Although the number of studies concerned with practice nurses were relatively few (8 out of the 77), they did relate to some of the most adventurous extensions of the role of community nursing.

It is already clear from this brief survey that some subject areas are better covered by studies than others and the reader can form his own judgement by referring back to the list of references for Chapter Four in which we have indicated those which relate to evaluative studies as we have defined them. We take up the issue of gaps in research in Chapter Six.

Year of publication

We identified 94 publications in all in relation to the 77 studies discussed in this chapter. The distribution of publications by year of publication is shown in Table 2.

The 'output' of publications appears to have built up to a peak in the years 1981-2 and to have declined somewhat in subsequent years. (The single publication included for 1986 reflects the fact that we stopped searching early in that year.)

A glance at the chart on pages 204-9 and references to Chapter Four suggest the following:
1) A high proportion of publications after 1983 were concerned with health visiting topics; we

seem to have identified very few for district
nursing after 1982.

2) Some topics, for example 'screening and surveillance of the elderly' (and indeed screening and surveillance of other age groups), are
spread over the whole period with which we are
concerned (1974 onwards). This may be partly
due to a sustained interest on the part of one
group of workers (see for example the studies
labelled A3.Al, 2,3 and B3. Al - and again in
the context of paediatric home nursing, the
publications relating to the study labelled
B4.1.)

3) Sometimes all the publications we have identified for inclusion in this chapter appeared
within a relatively short period - partly perhaps because of the passing popularity of the
subject under investigation (see for example
studies on health visiting services provided
out-of-normal working hours, publications
about all of which appeared in the years 1981-
2), or maybe because a substantial study appears to have answered most of the questions
being asked at that time (see for example publications relating to study B5.1 in the area
of day surgery and early discharge).

4) Sometimes the subject continues to be debated
without this interest apparently leading to
the undertaking of evaluative studies reflecting key issues in the debate - thus for example the issue of attachment versus geographical allocation of community nurses, about
which there were several studies in our chart
all published in or before 1979, has in the
1980s been the subject of lively controversy.

5) Some subject areas, in particular district
nurses in the treatment room and the work of
nurse practitioners, were not the subject of
any evaluative studies that fell within our
criteria during the period with which we are
concerned - though in the case of the latter,
evaluation of the work of one nurse practitioner (Barbara Stilwell) is about to be published.

Where reports of studies were published

The publication and/or publishing body are
listed in Table 3. Thirty-four of the 94 publications under discussion appeared in the nursing
press; 23 articles in the non-specific medical
press; 21 were published in the 'general health

services press' and eight were published in journals relating to particular clinical, technical or
client areas. Eight studies were assessed primarily on the basis of a research report.

Perhaps the most surprising absence is that of
anything from the Journal of Advanced Nursing.

Types of author
         The type(s) of author(s) could not be dis-
cerned in the case of six studies. Of the remaining 71, 24 studies involved nurses only as authors,
and nurses were involved as co-authors in a further
22 (by a nurse we mean someone with nursing qualifications). In the remaining 25 studies, nurses were
not involved as authors.

Among nurse authors, health visitors (excluding nursing officers) stood out as those most frequently involved as authors in studies, being involved in 28. Nursing officers (or above) were
involved as authors in 13 studies (some of the
nursing officers had health visitor qualifications
and/or district nursing qualifications). A district nurse author (other than nursing officer) was
involved in only three studies and a practice nurse
in only two studies. In four studies a nurse of
indistinguishable type was the author or one of the
authors.

Medically qualified authors were involved in
45 studies, general practitioners were involved in
21 of these, specialists in community medicine in
12, and other doctors (including hospital consultants) in 19. (Sometimes more than one 'type' of
medically qualified person was involved as author
in the same study.) Authors who were members of
social services departments were involved in three
studies, being the sole author in the case of one.

Research workers (including academic staff or
similar) who had neither nursing nor medical qualifications were involved as authors in 16 studies
and as sole author in two. In at least 35 studies,
at least one author was someone who might be expected to have had research training (included in
this group are persons we have labelled as academic
doctors, academic and research nurses, specialists
in community medicine, and academic and other research workers without nursing or medical qualifications).

Whilst the great majority of studies relating
to health visitors and most of those relating to
district nurses had one or more nurses among the
authors to publications, the small number of stud-

ies concerned with practice nursing and extending the role of nurses were relatively speaking much more likely not to have any nurses among their authors.

Location in which the study of the development was undertaken

All but two of the 77 studies were confined to one part of the country (see Table 4 - one of the two covering more than one part of the country was, however, entirely located within Wales). A relatively large number of studies were located in Scotland (21), most of the rest were in various parts of England apart from four in Wales and one in Northern Ireland. All but one of the studies located in the four Thames regional health authority areas were in the Greater London area. Overall 50 of the 77 studies took place in areas which we have classified as urban (including those in the Greater London area), three were in rural areas and all but one of the rest in 'mixed' areas. One study was consciously replicated in a rural area as well as in an urban area.

Characteristics of the evaluation reported

a) Design. Of the 77 studies, 11 were pilot or preliminary in some sense. Eighteen studies involved the use of controls (using the term loosely to denote a group of units with which the units subjected to the development under study were compared). One study involved the use of a mathematical model which served a similar function to a controlled study (under the assumptions of the model). In the case of most of the screening studies, it is arguable that a control group was not necessary in terms of the objectives (given that these related to the feasibility of the screening procedure and to the identification of medical, environmental and social problems of those approached previously not known to the health and social services). Even so this leaves at least 47 studies where controlled groups would have been helpful but were not employed - only nine of these 47 were described as preliminary or pilot studies.

The use of random samples, or random allocation between the groups subject to the development and the control group regime respectively, was in evidence for (at least part of) 14 studies. In a further 49, the units studied were the total number of cases or contacts receiving some service during a particular period (and in some cases a parallel group not receiving that service during the same or adjacent period). In the case of 14, it was either not clear on what basis the subjects were selected or, if it was, the subjects so chosen were neither the total population under consideration nor a random sample of that population.

In fact then, the clear majority of studies relied for information in a continuous series of cases or contacts located in a particular time period, or on the study of other groups of cases for which there was no apparently satisfactory rationale for their composition. In only six studies were controls and randomization both used in a manner akin to that customary for randomized controlled trials in clinical studies - and curiously all but one of these were published in or before 1982. Statistically speaking, straightforward experimental designs were used except in the case of study A3.B3 in which a crossover design (see page 188) was used.

b)   Scale of investigation. First we take as a crude measure of this, the size of the largest group of units (e.g. clients or contacts) considered in any part of a study. Eighteen of the studies involved consideration of 1,000 or more units (though sometimes in only a rather cursory fashion) while 16 involved less than 100 units - the remainder involved an intermediate number of units, the majority in the range 100-249 units). Most (11 out of 16) of the 'smallest' on our criterion for scale were not pilot studies and only two relied upon random sampling or allocation of units. (In very few studies of any size was use made of formal techniques of statistical inference, e.g. confidence intervals or significance tests - predictably in view of the fact that so few studies involved the use of random sampling or allocation techniques.)

As a second indicator we look at the number of sites or areas in which data were collected in the case of the part of the study involving the most widespread, in this sense, collection of data. About half the studies (36) were based on one or more sites of the following kind: a general (usually group) practice; practice(s) in a health centre; a primary health care team. In most cases (28) the study was based on just one such site. A small number were based on two or more such sites and one related in part to 39 primary health care teams.

Nine studies were based on (usually some part of) a hospital or clinic(s). The remaining studies were almost all based on areas; health districts (20) or part thereof (3), or some kind of local authority area (8). In almost all these cases it was just one such site (i.e. area).

Thus very infrequently was the field work replicated within a given study in more than one site. On the other hand, in some topic areas such as screening and surveillance of the elderly, a number of different studies did between them relate to programmes of screening and surveillance in a variety of circumstances - sometimes using a standard approach. Among these studies were several by the same authors, using approaches they had developed for this purpose, on various sites (see page 197).

c) <u>Costs of study</u>. In the case of five studies, information was given on the costs of the study, as distinct from implementing the development (see below).

<u>Information provided on input/output and outcome in relation to the development studied</u>
In 28 studies there was no explicit mention of costs or staff requirements. Virtually all of the studies, however, were in the nature of things concerned with giving details of the output of developments - cases treated, characteristics of cases etc. Generally speaking, studies concerned with developments in health visiting were rather less likely to mention costs and staff implications than those relating to other types of community nurse. Later studies were neither more nor less likely in general to mention costs and staff implications than earlier studies within our time period.

The outcome or consequences of the developments either in terms of the health and well-being of clients, or in terms of impact on that part of the health services providing the developments or any other part, was described in a subjective form in the case of 24 studies and not at all in three - it was not applicable in terms of the objectives in 13 - leaving 37 studies where information on outcome was based on something other than the opinions of clients or providers of the service. Once again, studies concerned with health visiting developments were less likely to provide 'hard' data on the outcome than those concerned with other kinds of community nurse.

Evaluative research on developments

This is not of course to undervalue in any way studies that made a point of seeking consumers' opinions about developments. In particular in 21 studies the development was appraised by among other things investigations into consumer satisfaction. This is in addition to those studies, mainly concerned with screening and surveillance of the elderly where clients were questioned in order to identify their needs for services, as distinct from their opinions about services or developments under study.

A note on surveys relating to community nursing which supplement or set in context information from evaluations of specific developments

A number of such surveys (for a definition of survey see page 188) have been published in and after 1974. In the references to this chapter, we have listed a number of those classified by topic as follows:

Organization of community nursing
Community nursing services out-of-normal working hours
Roles within and for community nursing
District nurses, practice nurses and the treatment room
The consumer viewpoint
Other

Each survey listed is marked according to the method of data collection used:
'Q' indicates that questionnaires were used to collect data (either by post or by interview);
'R' indicates that records were used for data. This includes both routine records and statistics as well as records specially kept (and sometimes specially designed too) for that particular survey, such as diaries or forms recording activities (possibly timed), characteristics of clients etc.

The surveys may have one of more of several purposes:
1) They may be investigations ranging widely over the field of community nursing, as it is at a particular point in time. Dunnell and Dobbs (1982) is a classic example of this type of survey and our frequent references to their work in Chapter Four is itself an acknowledgement of the value of their work in setting in context and understanding reports on a variety of developments.

202

2) They may have the purpose of reviewing on, say, a national basis the working of some particular facet or development in community nursing. A notable example of this is Harrisson et al. (1983) which gives a comprehensive picture, at the time of the enquiry, of district nursing and related caring services outside normal working hours in England and Wales in terms of costs, range of services provided and opinions of professionals on these services.

3) The primary purpose of the survey may be to obtain the opinions of a group of people, whether community nurses, other professionals, or clients or members of the general public on some particular issue or on community nursing services in general. (Surveys of type 1 and 2 above of course can include reference to the opinions of those approached, but we are thinking here of surveys in which the main aim is to obtain views possibly of a speculative nature on some development or issue, and any factual information collected primarily to form an understanding of these opinions, for example see Wiseman (1982) on professionals' views about the future of health visiting and Orr (1980) for a study of consumers' views on health visiting in Northern Ireland.

4) There is a further type of survey whose purpose is to obtain facts and informed opinions necessary to make predictions about future needs - we have listed several studies of this kind concerned with staffing levels.

CHART OF INFORMATION ON EVALUATIVE STUDIES DISCUSSED IN CHAPTER FIVE

(see pages 182-94 for abbreviations used)	Study No	Year	Journal or publisher	Author type(s)	Loc. of study Reg/c'try	Type of study	Pilot or prelim. study	Contr-olled trial	Random seln. or all'n	Units	Sites	Input	Outcome
HEALTH VISITING													
Organizational aspects of health visiting													
	A1.1	76	RR	RW	NS	L	N	N	?Y	120	2 HC	S	N
	A1.2	74	CETHV	D*,HV,RW	Various		N	N	Y/TE	50/ 5000	3 PHCT/ 36 PHCT	N*	NA
	A1.3	85	HV	NO,HV	SET	L	Y	NA	N	10	3 CL	S	Y
	A1.4	77	RR	NO*	SWT	L	N	N	TE	40/3000	1 HD	N	NA
	A1.5	79	HV	SCM	SET	L	N	Y	TE	3800	2 HD	N	NA
	A1.6	85	HV	HV	WM	M	N	N	N	20	1 HD	N	Su
Health visitors providing services	A2.1	(82	HSSJ	ANON)	NET	L	N	N	TE)	3100	1 HD	SC	Su) Co
		(81	HV	NO)					)	1100	1 HD	C	Su)
out of normal hours	A2.2	81	NT	HV	SWT	L	N	N	TE	160	1 HD	SC	Su
	A2.3	81	HV	NO	SW	U	N	N	TE	100	1 HD	SC	Su Co
	A2.4	81	NT	NO	NW	U	N	N	TE	200	1 HD	SC	Su
Health visitors and the elderly													
a)Health visitors and screening and surveillance of the elderly	A3.A1	76	JRCGP	GP*,HV	SCOT	U	?Y	NA	N	200	1 HC	'None' req'd	Su
	A3.A2	82	HB	GP*,HV	SCOT	U	N	Y	TE	120	1 GP	S	Y
	A3.A3	80	JRCGP	GP*,HV	SCOT	U	N	NA	Y	100	1 GP	N	NA
	A3.A4	84	NT	HV	EA	M	N	N	TE	230	1 GP	S	Su
	A3.A5	(74	NT	HV)	OX	U	N	N	TE	2000	1 LAD	SC	Su
		(75	HSSJ	NO,SCM,RW)									

(see pages 182-94 for abbreviations used)	Study No	Year	Journal or publisher	Author type(s)	Loc. of study Reg/c'try	Type of study	Pilot or prelim. study	Contr-olled trial	Random seln. or all'n	Scale Units	Sites	Input	Outcome
a) Health visitors and screening and surveillance of the elderly (cont'd)	A3.A6	74	BMJ	GP,NO,N	SCOT	U	N	N	TE	250	1 GP	S	NA
	A3.A7	75	AA	SCM	SCOT	M	N	N	TE	260	1 GP	S	Y
	A3.A8	75	NT	HV	YORKS	U	N	N	TE	220	1 HC	N	YSu
	A3.A9	85	HV	HV	SW	U	N?	N	TE	130	1 GP	N	YSu
	A3.A10	74	AA	HD,HV	SCOT	M	N	Y	Y	300	1 HC	N	Y
	A3.A11	84	HB	GP,NO,DN	SCOT	U	N	N	TE	900	1 GP	S	Su
	A3.A12	85	HV	NO	NI	M	N	N	TE	420	1 GP	N	YSu
b) Health visitors and the elderly - liaison and inter-vention schemes	A3.B1	83	RR	HV	SET	L	N?	N	Y	30	2 GP	N	NA Co
	A3.B2	84	MHVCN	HV	NW	U	N	N	N	50	1 GP	N	Y
	A3.B3	(81	NT	HV*	SCOT	U	N	Y	Y	60	1 GP	N	Y) Co
		(82	RCN	HV*	SCOT	U	N	Y	Y	60	1 GP	N	Y) Co
	A3.B4	84	BMJ	SCM,RW	W	U,R	N	Y	Y	1440	2 GP	YS	Y Co
Health visitors and family and child health care See also A7.1,A7.2	A4.1	(83	JRSS	RW)	TRENT	U	N	Y	TE	36000)	1 HD	S	Y
		(83	LA	RW,SCM,HV)						NS)			
		(84	MHVCN	SCM)						NS)			
	A4.2	84	HV	HV	SWT	U	Y	N	N	40	1 CL	S	Su Co
	A4.3	82	JECH	RW,D	W	U	Y	Y	N	140/440	1 HD	N	NA
	A4.4	86	HV	HV,PSYCH	W	M	N	Y	TE	40	1 DGH	N	YSu
Health visitors and psycho-social problems See also A4.4, A7.3	A5.1	(81	HV	HV)	NWT	L	N	Y	N	40	4 GP	N*	Su Co
		(82	BMJ	HV)									
	A5.2	80	NT	PN	WM	M	N	N	TE	60	1 GP	N	Su

(see pages 182-94 for abbreviations used)	Study No	Year	Journal or publisher	Author type(s)	Loc. of study Reg/c'try	Type of study	Pilot or prelim. study	Controlled trial	Random seln. or all'n	Scale n Units	Sites	Input	Information included on: Outcome
Health visitors liaising between hospital and community services	A6.1	(78 (82	HV NT	NO) NO)	NW	U	Y N	N	TE	670	1 H	N	Y Su
	A6.2	78	NT	HD*,HV	YORKS	U	N	N	N	50/100	1 H	S	Su
	A6.3	78	PH	HD,HV	TRENT	U	N	N	TE	2700	1 H	SC	Su
	A6.4	81	BMJ	HD*,HD,HV	SCOT	U	N	N	TE	230	1 H	N	YSu
	A6.5	84	NM	HV	NET	L	N	N	TE/TE	830/140	1 H/3 HD	S	Su
Specialization in health visiting	A7.1	(82 (82	CCHD	NS	NW	U	N	N	TE	(70 (60	SEVERAL) HD)	S?	Y Co
See also A4.4,A6.4	A7.2	81	HV	PSYCH	NW	M	N	N	N	5	NA	N	Su Co
	A7.3	81	HV	HV,HD,RW	N	M	N	N	TE	120	1 SECTOR of HD	S	Su
Health visitors and screening **a) Health visitors and the screening of infants and children. See also A4.1**	A8.A1	84	HB	SCM	SCOT	M	N	N	TE	800/220	1 HD	S	Y Co
	A8.A2	76	HB	SCM	SCOT	M	N	?Y	N	110/160	1 HD	N	N
	A8.A3	81	HB	SCM	SCOT	M	Y	N	TE	2600	1 HD	N	NA
b) Health visitors and the screening of adults (other than the elderly)	A8.B1	84	HV	HV	SW	M	N	N	TE	1100	2 GP	S	Su
	A8.B2	84	NT	HV	SWT	M	N	N	TE	800	1 GP	SC	YSu
	A8.B3	76	HB	GP,HV, CHEM	SCOT	U	N	N	TE	180	1 GP	SC	Y
DISTRICT NURSING Organizational aspects of district nursing	B1.1	77	RR	RW	WM	M	N	MM	Y/TE	40/2900	2 LAD	SC*	NA

See also A1.2,A1.4

(see pages 182-94 for abbreviations used)	Study No	Year	Journal or pub-lisher	Author type(s)	Loc. of study Reg/c'try	Type of study	Pilot or prelim. study	Contr-olled trial	Random seln. or all'n	Scale Units	Scale Sites	Input	Outcome
District nurses providing services out-of-hours	B2.1	80	HB	GP,RW	SCOT	M	N	N	TE	30/110	Pt HD	SC	Su
	B2.2	81	BMJ	SCM,D	NET	L	N	N	TE	30/240	1 LB	SC	YSu
District nurses and the elderly a)District nurses and the screening and surveillance of the elderly See also A3.A8	B3.A1	76	HB	GP*,HV	SCOT	R	N	NA	TE	150	ONE ISLAND	N	NA
	B3.A2	82	HV	N,GP,HD	SW	M	Y	Y	N	280	1 GP/LAD	S	Y
	B3.A3	75	NPHT	N*	WM	U	Y	N	Y	130	1 GP	S	Su
	B3.A4	75	NM	DN	SCOT	U	N	N	TE	290	1 GP	N	Su
b)Liaison and inter-vention schemes See also B9.2	B3.B1	82 (84	RR) NT)	GP,RW	EA	R	N	Y	TE	40/1500	12 VILL-AGES 1GP	SC*	Y Co
	B3.B2	80	AA	NS	SCOT	U	Y	N	TE?	30	1 GP	S	Su Co
	B3.B3	82	BMJ	HD,NO,SS	N	U	?Y	N	N	10/20	Pt HD	SC	Y
	B3.B4	77	BMJ	D*	WM	U	N	N	N	130	1 HD	SC	Su
Paediatric home nursing See also B9.3	B4.1	(75 (80 (85	NT) JPS) BMJ)	NS) NS) NS)	WESS	U	N	N	TE	(630/ (12000 (	1 HD	SC	YSu
	B4.2	77	BMJ	HD,SCM, GP*,RW	N	U	Y	N	TE	60	1 HD	N	YSu Co
Day surgery and early discharge	B5.1	78(3) 80	BJS, JECH(2)) NT)	HD,SCM GP*,RW	SCOT	U	N	Y	Y	360 110	1 HD	SC	Y Co
	B5.2	77	LA	NS	N	U	N	Y	Y	60/120	1 H	SC	Y Co

(see pages 182-94 for abbreviations used)	Study No	Year	Journal or publisher	Author type(s)	Loc. of study Reg/c'try	Type of study	Pilot or prelim. study	Contr-olled trial	Random seln. or all'n	Units	Sites	Input	Outcome
Intensive home nursing See also B3.B2, B3.B3	B7.1)	82	BMJ	(GP,SS)					(	50	1 HD	SC*)	
	)	82	RR	(	EA	U	N		N (	50	1 HD	SC*)	YSu Co
	)	85	JDN	NO)					(	900	1 HD	SC*)	
Nursing and related care - joint schemes with social services	B9.1	81	HSSJ	SS	SW/WESS	M	N	N	TE	200	1 C	SC	YSu
	B9.2	82	RR	NS	NET	L	N	N	TE	70/660	1 SECTION of 1 LB	S	Y
	B9.3	81	HSSJ	NS	WESS	M	Y	N	TE	210	3 LAD	SC	YSu Co
Support services for community nurses in the care of the dying	B10.1	81	LA	HD,N,RW	SET	L	N	N	TE	670	1 H	S	YSu
	B10.2	(82	JRCGP	D)	SCOT	U	N	N	TE	220	1 LAD	S	Y
		(80	PRACT	D)									
	B10.3	80	PGMJ	D*	SET	L	N	Y	TE	20/50	2 LB	C	YSu Co
Support for district nurses from specialist and liaison nurses, and from other services	B11.1	81	RR	NO*	NWT	L	Y	N	TE	130/70	1 HOSP	S	Su

Other district nursing See A5.2 and A8.B2

(see pages 182–94 for abbreviations used)	Study No	Year	Journal or publisher	Author type(s)	Loc. of study Reg/c'try	Type of study	Pilot or prelim. study	Contr-olled trial	Random seln. or all'n	Units	Sites	Input	Outcome
PRACTICE NURSES													
The practice nurse's work in the treatment room	C2.1	74	HB	GP	SCOT	U	N	N	TE	2000	1 HC	S	Y
	C2.2	(80	BMJ	GP,SCM)	TRENT	M	N	N	TE	61000	1 GP	N	NA
		(81	BMJ	GP,SCM)						102000			
Extensions of the role of the	C3.1	79	JRCGP	GP,RW	SWT	L	N	Y	Y/TE	40/10000	1 GP	SC	YSu Co
practice nurse	C3.2	83	BMJ	GP,PN,RW	W	R	N	N	TE	50	1 GP	S	Y Co
See also A5.2	C3.3	81	JRCGP	GP	WM	M	N	N	TE	3000	1 GP	N	N
EXTENDING THE ROLE OF THE NURSE													
Miscellaneous ex-	D2.1	76	HB	GP*,RW	SCOT	U	N	Y	TE	50/100	1 GP	N	Y
tensions of the nurse's role	D2.2	82	JECH	GP	TRENT	M	N	Y	Y	290	1 GP	N	NA
Attitudes towards extending the nurse's role See also C3.1	D3.1	76	CH	GP,RW	N	U	N	N	TE/Y	3100, 400	1 GP	S	Y Co

Table 1

Subjects with which the studies were concerned

Subject of study	Type of health services staff with which primarily concerned	No. of studies
Organization of community nursing	Health visitors	4
	District nurses	1
	Both health visitors and district nurses	2
Provision of community nursing services out-of normal working hours	Health visitors	4
	District nurses	2
Screening and surveillance (a) Elderly	Health visitors	11
	District nurses	4
	Both Health visitors and district nurses	1
(b) Adults (i.e. not confined to elderly)	Health visitors	3 (1)
	District nurses and health visitors	1
(c) Infants and children	Health visitors	4 (2)
Health visitors and family and child health care (excluding screening and surveillance)	Health visitors	6 (3)
	District nurses	2
Paediatric home nursing	Health visitors	4
Liaison and intervention schemes for elderly	District nurses	5 (4)

Table 1 (Cont.)

Subject of study	Type of Health Services staff with which primarily concerned	No. of studies
Nurses and related care – joint schemes with social services	District nurses	3(5)
Psycho-social problems	Health visitors	3 (6)
	Health visitors, district nurses, practice nurses	1 (7)
Specialization in health visiting	Health visitors	3 (8)
Liaising between hospital and) community)	Health visitors	5
	District nurses	1
Day surgery and early discharge	District nurses	2
Intensive home nursing	District nurses	3 (9)
Support services for community nurses in the care of the dying	District nurses	3
Treatment room activities	Practice nurses	2
Extending role of community nurses	Health visitors, district nurses	
	practice nurses	2 (10)
	Practice nurses	4
	Health visitors	1 (11)

Note: some studies relate to more than one subject and appear more than once in this table, in particular:

(1) Includes 1 counted also under Extending role of community nurses (health visitors)

(2) Includes 1 counted also under Health visitors and family and child health

(3) Includes 2 counted also under Specialization in health visiting and 1 under Psycho-social problems (health visitors)

(4) Includes 1 counted also under Nursing and related care – joint schemes with social services and 2 under Intensive home nursing

(5) Includes 1 counted also under Liaison and intervention schemes for the elderly (district nurses)

(6) Includes 1 counted also under Health visiting and family and child health problems and 1 counted also under Specialization in health visiting

(7) Includes 1 counted also under Extending role of community nurses

(8) Includes 2 counted also under Health visitors and family and child health and 1 counted also under Psycho-social problems (health visitors)

(9) Includes 2 counted also under Liaison and intervention schemes for the elderly (district nurses)

(10) Includes 1 counted also under Psycho-social problems (health visitors, district nurses, practice nurses)

(11) Includes 2 counted also under Screening and surveillance of adults (health visitors)

Evaluative research on developments

Table 2

Analysis of publications by year of publication

Year of Publication	No. published that year
1974	5
1975	6
1976	7
1977	5
1978	6
1979	2
1980	9
1981	17
1982	16
1983	4
1984	10
1985	6
1986	1
All publications	94

Table 3

Analysis of publications by journal or other place
of publication

Where published	No. of publications
The nursing press	
Nursing Times	12
Nursing Mirror	2
Health Visitor	15
Journal of Community Nursing (Journal of District Nursing)	1
Council for the Education and Training of Health Visitors	1
Royal College of Nursing	1
Midwife, Health Visitor and Community Nurse	2
Non-specific medical press	
British Medical Journal	13
The Lancet	3
Postgraduate Medical Journal	1
Journal of the Royal College of General Practitioners	5
The Practitioner	1
General health services press	
Health and Social Service Journal	4
Health Bulletin	10
Public Health	1
Nuffield Provincial Hospitals Trust	1
Croom Helm	1
Journal of Epidemiology and Community Health	4
Journals concerned with particular clinical technical or client areas	
Child Care Health and Development	2
Age and Ageing	3
British Journal of Surgery	1
Journal of Pediatric Surgery	1
Journal of the Royal Statistical Society	1
Research reports	8
TOTAL NUMBER OF PUBLICATIONS	94

Table 4

The locations in which studies of developments were
undertaken

Location of study	No. of studies
English Regional Health Authorities	
N E Thames	4
S E Thames	5
S W Thames	5
N W Thames	2
An unstated Thames Region	1
Northern	5
Yorkshire	2
Trent	4
East Anglia	3
Wessex	3*
Oxford	1
South Western	5*
West Midlands	6
Mersey	0
North Western	5
Northern Ireland	1
Scotland	21
Wales	4
Various	1
TOTAL NUMBER OF STUDIES	77

* One study took place at locations in the Wessex
and South Western Regions

Chapter Six

IDENTIFYING THE PRIORITIES FOR FUTURE RESEARCH

INTRODUCTION

What further research is needed into community
nursing? To help answer this question, we drew
upon the three main sources of information used
throughout this book. These have been: the views
of chief nursing officers in England who responded
to a postal survey; the views of representatives of
professional organizations and of some leading members of the professions; and the views expressed in
the extensive literature on developments in community nursing. In looking at the literature and at
the research which has been done, we have also
formed our own views about the priorities for future research.

From these various sources, some consensus
emerged about the priorities for future research
and these priorities are now discussed in this
chapter.

The areas we have finally identified for future research are:

Management structures in community nursing
Attachment versus geographical deployment of
    community nurses
Roles of community nurses
    - the role of the health visitor
    - the role of the district nurse and
        nurse practitioner
    - the role of the specialist community
        nurse
    - the role of the district nurse in
        relation to the practice nurse
Out-of-hours services provided by district
    nurses

Identifying the priorities for future research

MANAGEMENT STRUCTURES IN COMMUNITY NURSING

What is the best way of organizing the management of community nursing?
Does the 'best way' vary between different
types of districts?
What should the managerial relationship be
between community nurses
         - and general practitioners
         - and senior nurses
         - and the health authority?
How autonomous/independent should community
nurses be in carrying out their work?

An issue which was given high priority for
research by a number of professional bodies (including the CETHV, RCGP, GMSC and RCN) and persons
approached, and by ourselves, was the management
structure of community nursing. District nurses
and health visitors work, at least in theory, in
primary health care teams with general practitioners. However, the doctors are independent and equal
(apart from the constraints of a group practice or
a senior partner) whereas the nurses are part of a
managerial hierarchy within the district health
authority. With the implementation of the recommendations of the National Health Service Management Inquiry (1983) and the advent of non-nursing
managers, dissatisfaction among nurses has increased. The Standing Medical Advisory Committee and
the Standing Nursing and Midwifery Advisory Committee (1981) reported difficulties arising between
general practitioners and nursing officers over the
attachment of nursing staff, and over the difference in expectations as to which tasks nursing
staff should undertake. (See Chapters Two and Three
for more detail on this, the Harding Committee
Report.) These difficulties in recent years have
coincided with an increasing sense of professional-
ism among nurses and a desire for more independence. Hockey (1984) wrote in relation to practice
nurses:

In my view all nursing staff should have the
same employer and this employer should be the
health authority and not the general practitioner. I believe that nurses and doctors
should work together in a collegiate rather
than an employee/employer relationship. For
such a system to operate effectively, the nursing staff must be competent and be allowed to

217

work as professional people, judging for themselves under what conditions they can and
should undertake particular and professional
nursing functions. Only nurses who can be
trusted to act independently in a professionally responsible manner should be employed as
health visitors, district nurses or practice
nurses.

There have been suggestions as to what form
alternative management arrangements might take, and
these were mentioned in Chapter Four in the part
'Ideas for future developments'. The report of the
Community Nursing Review (DHSS 1986) identified a
number of management problems in community nursing,
including the remoteness of managers from staff in
primary health care teams, the separation of district nursing and health visitor management and a
lack of sensitivity to the needs of the individuals
forming the community. The cornerstone of the review's solution to these problems was the establishment of neighbourhood nursing services, each managed by a neighbourhood nursing manager, who would
retain some clinical responsibilities. The population served by the neighbourhood nursing service -
about 10,000 to 25,000 patients - is intended to be
sufficiently small to prevent remoteness in management and to foster integrated services. The review
also recommended that an agreement about services
provided be signed by general practitioners and
nursing managers, which could resolve problems in
that area. As far as we know there has been no
research into alternative kinds of management arrangements for community nurses, unlike the other
areas of research priority which we identify.
(Though as this book goes to press, we understand
that neighbourhood nursing services are being tried
out on an experimental basis in Brighton Health
District (Chairman, Mrs J Cumberlege who was the
Chairman of the Community Nursing Review Team
(DHSS, 1986). This lack of research is one reason
for giving the subject a high priority, in addition
to the problems which the current arrangements give
rise to. The consultations we had with
representatives of professional organizations and
others have confirmed that there is an a priori
case for examining the way in which community nurses are managed with a view to finding improvements
if possible.
    The first stage for any research is arguably
to establish whether the problems identified are

widespread and, if so, over what kinds of issues
and in what kinds of circumstances the problems
particularly manifest themselves. This implies
undertaking suitable surveys of interested parties.
In the case of management structures these parties
comprise attached community nurses, general practitioners to whom community nurses are attached, and
nursing officers with line responsibilities for
attached community nurses. The surveys would take
into account various factors such as type of area -
whether urban or rural - the way in which community
services relate to the unit structure of the district, type of general practice in the area, the
qualifications of the nursing officers in relation
to the staff they manage and so on. Respondents
might also be asked to comment on alternative arrangements for organizing community nurses within
primary health care teams such as have been sket-
ched above and in pages 176-78. The views of clients might also be sought about existing arrangements.
    The next stage, supposing that the first stage
did indeed indicate that there were problems needing attention, would be to formulate plausible alternative arrangements and to try them out on an
experimental basis in a suitable variety of circumstances. The service costs (that is the costs apart
from those of undertaking research itself in such
experimentation) need be minimal. It is possible
that some models for the relationship between nursing officer and attached community nursing staff,
such as those Kratz and we have proposed (see pages
176-78) could, by freeing the nursing officer from
some of her managerial responsibilities, leave time
for her to develop her role as a channel of communication on DHSS and health authority policy and as
an educator of her field staff - making fuller and
more creative use of her nursing experience than
would be possible as a straight-forward line-
manager.

ATTACHMENT VERSUS GEOGRAPHICAL DEPLOYMENT OF
COMMUNITY NURSES

    Is attachment necessarily always the best way
of organizing community nurses?
    -    Is it economic?
    -    Does it provide the best service for
         patients?
    -    Is it an efficient way of using trained
         staff?

Identifying the priorities for future research

Do the advantages of being attached and thus belonging to a primary health care team outweigh the disadvantages?
What modifications to organizational arrangements could be made to reduce the problems of attachment?

In contrast to the area of management structures in community nursing, there has been a certain amount of research over the years, though not much recently, into the attachment of community nurses to general practices, a development now long established and widely adopted. However, difficulties with it have been reported and some health authorities have recently reverted to a geographical system of deployment.

Serious problems with attachment schemes were identified by, amongst others, the Harding Committee (1981), the Acheson Report (1981) and the Health Visitors' Association (1981) - reports which are discussed in Chapter Three, see pages 80, 82 and 74 respectively. The Community Nursing Review (DHSS, 1986) recognized that problems could occur when 'the practice population and the health authority population do not match up' and favoured the idea of general practitioners adopting 'zones' for their patients. However, the review body felt that their recommended system of neighbourhood nursing services would resolve problems of geographical and attached schemes in general practice, and that the matter tended 'to get blown up out of proportion'. The review, in recommending that an agreement be signed by general practitioners and nursing managers about services the nurses in the primary care team should provide, hoped to improve teamwork in general practice. Respondents to our survey of chief nursing officers wanted research into this area, in particular into the value of attachment schemes compared to a geographical system in terms of benefit to the patient and of cost effectiveness. Representatives of the CETHV, RCGP, GMSC and RCN also saw this area as a high priority for research. Despite the long established practice of attachment, discussion in the literature on the effects, and the merits or otherwise of attachment schemes, still continues.

Those who question the merits of attachment argue that it can be uneconomic compared with the 'geographical patch' approach especially in inner city areas. In these areas a large number of community nurses (using this collectively to refer to

health visitors and district nurses) may be working
in the same locality and a particular nurse's travelling time is increased because her patients are
scattered over a relatively large area, either
viewed in horizontal terms or in the case of high-
rise flats, vertically speaking. Attachment in
these circumstances also means that no one community nurse has an overall responsibility (within
her sphere of activities) for a given geographical
patch, thus no one has a duty or indeed the capacity to know what is going on in the patch, for
instance to follow up unregistered patients or to
build up a network of contacts which would enable
her to get early warning of problems occurring
within some families. There is, it is argued, a
great deal of difference between being a district
nurse or health visitor for a particular small locality, and having a similar role in respect of the
patients of a couple of general practitioners,
scattered over the community. Several of the studies reported in Chapter Four (see pages 113-14,
116, 141-42) compared the effects of community
nurses working on attached and other bases. The
conclusions of these, which at the risk of repet-
ition are gathered together below, are less dramatic and conclusive than the vigour of the debate
on this subject might suggest.

Poulton (1977), comparing aligned and attached
health visitors and district nurses in the Wandsworth and East Merton Health District, concluded
that:

> there is a significant difference in the work-
> ing pattern of health visitors who are attach-
> ed and those who are aligned. The main diff-
> erences are:
> 1. The aligned* health visitors spend more
>   time on client visits including routine
>   visits.
> 2. The attached* health visitors spend more

---

*'Nurses practising and working with GPs from hea-
lth centres or group practices are called "attachments"; nurses working with a number of GPs in various practices but based at centres are called "alignment". In addition to these schemes some health
visitors and home nurses serve a geographical district in order to cope with the drifters in the
population who are not registered with a GP.
(Poulton, 1977)

> time in consultation with the general practitioner.
> The home nurse ... also shows a significant variation of working patterns between schemes throughout almost all aspects of her work. The main differences are:
> 1. The attached nurse spends less time on visiting patients at home but compensates for it by carrying out care at the surgery.
> 2. The aligned nurse and nurses engaged on relief work, spend more time on travelling than their colleagues.

Walsworth-Bell (1979) compared the work of health visitors in two districts, Greenwich and Bexley, and concluded that:

> There seems a common core of health visiting practice ... which is untouched by how the health visitor's work is organized ... However the differences should not be minimized. The advantages for attached health visitors are that they seem more approachable to clients and their clinics are used for more informal consultations. The advantages for geographical health visitors are the higher number of "no-one initiated" visits, and increased follow-up of families known not to have a GP.'

Dawtrey (1976), examining the work of health visitors in two health centres in Inner London, found that the breadth of cases presented to a health visitor was influenced by whether she was attached or unattached but concluded that both approaches had distinctive contributions to make to the care provided to a community.

Dunnell and Dobbs (1982), in their survey of community nurses in 24 health districts, also produced some information about attachment. It was found that for district nurses, midwives and health visitors, not being attached to general practice and working with a large number of practices were related to a less positive assessment on their part of relationships with general practice. However assessments in relation to patient-related aspects of their work 'were not related to patterns of attachment and patchworking, nor to the number of practices worked with ...'. There was a slight tendency for attached nurses to view the amount of travel they did as excessive. When information about actual travelling time from the diaries was compared, there were no differences between attached and not attached district nurses, midwives and health visitors.

Clark (1981), who reviewed thirteen studies comparing characteristics of the work of health visitors organized on attached and geographical patch bases respectively, concluded that:

a) the differences reported are small, and
b) such differences as are found cannot be conclusively attributed to (the presence or absence of) attachment'.

However, a study comparing district nurses working on attached and geographical bases respectively, in part of one Midlands area health authority (West Midlands Regional Health Authority, Management Services Division, 1977) warned against the danger of taking these methods of working at their face value. It appears that in the town where a complete attachment scheme was formally in operation, this was not rigidly adhered to; nor was it the case that in the town where nurses were organized on a geographical basis that this entirely determined their method of working. 'In both towns there was evidence of work sharing to reduce pressure in certain areas and to reduce travelling time and costs.' Hence it was thought that the above analysis could not be expected to identify differences between true attachment and true geographical patch schemes. In fact in the conclusions based on an actual study of the nurses working according to the two approaches, very little difference was found. The authors tried, therefore, to compare the costs of district nurses working on an attached and geographical basis by means of the analysis of theoretical models incorporating the central characteristics respectively of the two approaches. They concluded that if one accepts the assumptions built into these models, geographical allocation would be considerably less expensive than attachment.

Dingwall and Watson (1980) argue that, at least in the present system of primary health care, which has changed in recent years, attachment should not be abandoned hastily. They recommend a series of trials to evaluate attached versus district systems.

Identifying the priorities for future research

Clearly questions remain to be answered in this area. What seems to be lacking is reliable information about the circumstances in which attachment, geographical allocation and various intermediate alternatives work well and badly. A suitably extensive survey could provide the answers. In the light of this knowledge it should then be possible to select and try out under as near as possible experimental conditions a short list of potential 'best buys' for particular situations.

ROLES OF COMMUNITY NURSES

The role of the health visitor
Is there a role for the health visitor?
Should the roles of health visitors and district nurses be modified, particularly in relation to one another?
Should e.g. the roles of health visitor and district nurse or health visitor and social worker be combined
- generally/nationwide?
- in some places only?

The role of the health visitor has been the subject of considerable research but despite this there is a call for still more, as a number of issues are unresolved or have emerged recently.

Respondents to our survey of chief nursing Officers in England thought there was a need for research into this area. A number of professional organisations, including the Health Visitors' Association, the Council for the Education and Training of Health Visitors, the Royal College of General Practitioners, the General Medical Services Committee, and the Royal College of Nursing, thought that the role of the health visitor, and the relationship between her roles and the roles of others such as the district nurse and the school nurse, was a matter for priority in research. The Health Visitors' Association has called for a national enquiry into the proper role and functions of, and the relationship between, health visitors and school nurses (Editorial, 1982). The Association pointed out in support of this call that there had been many changes in the characteristics of the population served by health visitors and school nurses since the last enquiry into health visiting, with some reference to school nursing, was carried out in 1956 by the Jameson Committee (Ministry of Health, 1956). Yet the calculations and recommendations of the Jameson Committee are still used, the Association stated, as a basis for assessing the acceptable ratio of health visitors to populations served. The development of primary health care teams with the basing of health visitors' case loads on patient lists instead of on geographical areas has also had a profound effect on health visiting and school nursing. To a considerable extent this has meant that health visiting has become more and more divorced from school nursing, and training specifically designed for school nurses has emerged. Prior to 1974,

> Whilst working as local government officers health visitors claimed and were given the status of practitioners in their own right. Within the nursing hierarchy of the integrated NHS this status is proving incompatible with the type of managerial and financial control required by health authorities, and increasingly professional judgements are becoming the subject of challenge and even of disciplinary action.
> Another real anxiety (to the Health Visitors' Association) is the growing number of small surveys or simply expressions of opinion about health visiting and school nursing which are influencing health authorities and others often quite unjustifiably .... In addition to the many other reasons for a full scale enquiry it is naturally of great concern to the Association that the future development of health visiting and school nursing should be based on fully informed opinion resulting from a nation-wide enquiry, and not on one or more of a variety of limited surveys which may not be scientifically designed and which cover only a restricted geographical area.'
> (Editorial, 1982).

Hicks (1976) has argued that there was a case for combining the role of health visitor and district nurse, and took the health service professions to task for their unwillingness to even contemplate let alone experiment with such changes.

The Community Nursing Review (DHSS, 1986) felt that health visitors and district nurses were 'trapped by tradition' in their ways of working. They thought that the problem would be solved by the establishment of the neighbourhood nursing services recommended in their report as the 'professional demarcation lines of responsibility which have existed for so long would fade at last', and wanted more training in common for community nurses.

Goodwin (1982) felt that there should be an enquiry into health visiting which should 'examine and make recommendations about the proper role, and functions of the health visitor and to establish up to date health visitor-to-population ratios in the light of changes in the health visitor's work necessitated by altered patterns of health, and social conditions'. Among the questions she felt that any enquiry should try to answer were:

- What is the evidence that the health visitor's work has any effect?
- What do consumers think of the service?
- Is a nursing background, and existing training, the most appropriate training for health visitors?
- Are health visitors necessary or has some other kind of worker more potential for prevention?

The discussion document 'Thinking About Health Visiting' (RCN, 1983) concluded that health visiting is nursing, and set out a number of problems and questions for the profession to address itself to in connection with the role of health visiting in the future; see in particular pages 85 and 86 of this book. (In addition, a number of suggestions which have been made about the roles of health visitors are referred to in Chapter Four in the part entitled 'Ideas for future developments').

Thus there is a continuing discussion in the literature about the role of the health visitor, despite the amount of research completed and ongoing in this area. However, much of the research done (and referred to in the relevant parts of Chapter Four) has been of a survey type, and not experimental, and there is a dearth of research into some aspects of the health visitor's role. In particular although there appears to have been a considerable growth in the number of specialized health visitors and liaison health visitors, there has been little research into these developments (see below).

Even in an area central to the health visitor's role, namely child assessment, there has been a relatively recent call (arising out of a survey of health authority policy and practice by Connolly

(1982)) for an examination as to where they can most effectively contribute in this work.

Of course the role of the health visitor cannot be looked at in isolation from the roles of other staff, in particular school nurses and social workers, but also district nurses. Studies concerned with the role of the health visitor and other community nurses jointly have been lacking, although some research is now in progress in this field at the Polytechnic of the South Bank (and the Centre for the Study of Primary Care in Tower Hamlets).

The role of the district nurse and nurse practitioner

By contrast with the health visitor, developments in the role of the district nurse appeared to be less contentious, partly perhaps because details of organization and role assignment apart, the need for suitably trained persons to give nursing care in the community is not in dispute. The question is 'in what ways should her role be developed if at all?' One possibility would be for a district nurse to take on the screening and educational functions associated with health visitors in the case of elderly persons. The adoption of the nursing process approach in district nursing, with its implication of greater autonomy in devising and managing the conventional nursing activities for district nursing sisters and the direct conveyance of nursing plans so developed to hospital nurses where patients are admitted (and vice versa on discharge) is another area of development. There has also been a suggestion that the district nursing team (taking this to include the district nursing sister, other trained nurses – SRN and SEN – and nursing auxiliaries) should be responsible for care of patients in greater depth, taking account of all their social and other circumstances in their management in the nursing sense of the case.

The proposal by the Community Nursing Review Team (DHSS, 1986) that there should be nurse practitioners in neighbourhood nursing teams implies a very different kind of organizational setting for such workers than has been reported on so far, and arguably calls for careful monitoring of pilot schemes to explore amongst other things the implications of a nurse practitioner working in a team led by a neighbourhood nursing manager and the impact on the work of others in the team, particularly health visitors and district nurses.

The role of the specialist community nurse

What specialties should there be in community nursing?

What should be the role of the specialist community (or hospital) nurse in relation to other community nursing staff?

Just as health visitor specialists have developed so have district nurse specialists, and the role of the specialist nurse, particularly where based outside the primary health care team setting, was a matter of concern, especially to the RCN and other nursing professional organizations, and some other nursing respondents whom we consulted. There was a feeling that it was best for the 'outsider' specialist nurses to train community nurses rather than supplant them in providing specialist care for patients directly. In the consultations with the professional organizations, there was also widespread support for the idea that community nurses should develop specialist interests and skills and receive suitable training for this purpose, whilst remaining within their community setting, and that the local groups of colleagues with whom they were associated would then be able to look to them as a resource for specialist information and advice, even though they continue to practice as generic health visitors or district nurses for at least part of the time themselves.

Problems arising from the emergence of specialist nurses were also identified by the Community Nursing Review Team (DHSS, 1986). They thought the problems arose particularly when a specialist nurse was based in a hospital, and providing 'nursing care and advice in people's homes without prior consultation with district nurses or health visitors causing confusion for the client and unnecessary friction between hospital and community services'. The review team did not question the development of specialist nurses, but recommended that as far as possible they should be based in the community, and managed as part of the neighbourhood nursing service. 'They should aim to co-ordinate their work with neighbourhood nurses and other care agencies' and should help community nurses to develop their own expertise.

We think that research into the types and roles of specialist nursing staff working in the community, who have emerged in a very 'ad hoc' way, is now a high priority.

The role of the district nurse in relation to the practice nurse

How best should the work of the district nurse and the practice nurse be arranged in relation to each other?

Does open access to a nurse at the surgery ultimately provide a better outcome for the patient?

The role of the district nurse also has to be considered in relation to the role of the practice nurse, and although there was little call for research in this area, except for some interest from the RCN and the RCGP, we feel that the it needs some further investigation, as practice nurses are now an established group of staff in primary health care.

The Community Nursing Review (DHSS, 1986) recommended that 'subsidies to general practitioners enabling them to employ staff to perform nursing duties should be phased out'. The review was against the employment of practice nurses by general practitioners, as the arrangements for reimbursement 'give very uncertain value for money' and because nurses 'should not be subject to control and direction by doctors over their professional work'. The review thought that the systems of neighbourhood nursing services and written agreements between nursing services and general practitioners, would mean that there would be less reason or need for general practitioners to employ their own nurses, since community nurses could take on new roles in collaboration with general practitioners.

However, the discussion paper 'Primary Health Care' (DHSS et al. 1986) states that the government will continue to reimburse general practitioners to employ practice nurses. Studies of the work of practice nurses and district nurses suggest that practice nurses are more likely to undertake technical activities of the sort normally associated with general practitioners than district nurses who undertake more of the caring aspects of the job. This is partly because practice nurses are mainly accountable to the general practitioner, who will refer any patient to the practice nurse that he thinks fit. The district nurse has to work within the confines of the policy laid down by the health authority and there is in particular the possible difficulty of the district nurse feeling that some referrals from the general practitioner to herself are inappropriate for someone employed by another authority, particularly where the general practitioner obtains a fee for the item of service although actually performed by a district nurse. Certainly there seems to be a need for experiments about approaches to co-ordinating the work of practice nurses and district nurses, and towards the evolving of a policy generally applicable to family doctors as to how services associated with the two kinds of nurse can be appropriately provided.

Of course the relationship between the role of the district nurse and the role of the practice nurse could be affected by changes in the management arrangements for community nurses generally, an area which we have recommended above as having a high priority for research.

If the question of role commands wide interest among the people and organizations consulted and the literature read, it must also in terms of time have a claim to being among the first topics studied. It could be argued that until the question of roles is settled, there is little point, except as a stop gap measure in committing resources, in studying staffing levels of existing types of staff. The argument here rests on the expectation, not so much that research on roles is likely to produce new and radically different types of nurse in the community, but that the allocation of border-line and new tasks as between existing and/or possibly new types of community nursing staff is likely to have a substantial effect on staffing levels required for the various types of nursing staff in question. This of course is only one way of looking at the problem which could be turned on its head. For example, given the existing and projected staff levels in health visiting, district nursing and other categories of community nurse, the research question asked might be what functions should they be given (or is it reasonable to expect them to carry out) and what extra tasks could be allocated to each staff type. Thus there is a real Pandora's box of inter-related and often controversial issues associated with the study of the roles of community nurses.

OUT-OF-HOURS SERVICES PROVIDED BY DISTRICT NURSES

What is the best way of organizing out-of-hours services, e.g. night sitters, tucking down

services etc.?
What is the best way of organizing services
- to be cost-effective?
- to provide an adequate service?
What sort of services do patients and relatives prefer?
What is the cost-effectiveness of providing out-of-hours services in the community compared to admitting patients to an institution?

Evening and night nursing services provided by district nurses, 'night sitters' and nursing auxiliaries have become widespread. The need for these services is not questioned, judging from the literature, interviews with representatives of medical and nursing professions, and our survey of chief nursing officers. The provision of a 24-hour nursing service was regarded by the Community Nursing Review Team (DHSS, 1986) as a minimum service which should be provided by each health authority in order 'to reduce admission to hospital and to enhance quality of care'. Neither were these services seen, in general, as needing to be researched. However, there are important unanswered questions about these services, which we feel, as did some respondents to the CNO survey, need research.

A major national survey of out-of-hours services provided by district nurses has been reported on by Harrisson and colleagues (1983). The study included surveys of chief nursing officers, district nurses and general practitioners. It presents a comprehensive picture of current practice and professional views upon out-of-hours nursing services in England and Wales. (See page 142 of this book.) The authors, however, suggested that further research was required in two areas:

a) A survey of patients receiving out-of-hours services, including the views and experience they and their relatives had of the service.
b) An in-depth investigation in a limited number of districts of different types of out-of-hours services to provide data for assessing optimum staffing patterns (i.e. the mix of staff with various levels of training in different types of districts.)

Hardly any in-depth studies of specific out-of-hours schemes were in fact found in our search of the literature, although there were a number of descriptions of schemes. The studies and schemes reported demonstrated a variety of types of out-of-hours nursing services. These included a nurse staying all night with the patient; a night sitter (that is an unqualified person given some training and employed by health or social services) staying all night, with a nurse on call or making routine visits during the night; and a 'tucking down' service where the nurse comes in to settle the patients at night. Obviously, as Harrisson et al. (1983) describe, these variations have different cost implications, depending on the type of staff used (qualified or not) and how much they are with one patient or with several during any given evening or night. One study (Martin and Ishino, 1981) concluded that providing evening and night nursing services was less costly than institutional care except for Part III accommodation. Not that this was a realistic option as the patients in question were too ill or handicapped to be accepted for Part III accommodation.

Another factor to be taken into account is whether or not providing out-of-hours services keeps at home patients who would otherwise have to go into institutional care, and for how long. A number of the schemes described in the literature asserted that patients were able to stay at home by using these services, but there was no real proof of this. If keeping patients at home and out of hospital is an objective of providing out-of-hours community nursing services, then this needs to be demonstrated.

The views and experiences (including costs of various kinds borne - money, time, etc.) of patients and their relatives or other lay carers on this particular matter are of importance too.

Respondents to our survey of chief nursing officers, who wanted research in this field, were interested in the cost-effectiveness of providing out-of-hours services in the community compared to admitting patients to an institution, the cost-effectiveness of the various mixes of types of staff providing the services, and the needs of patients receiving the service.

IN CONCLUSION

Any list of research priorities must (a) be of arbitrary length and (b) necessarily run the risk of early obsolescence as with time new projects are commissioned and new problems come and old ones disappear with changing circumstances.

After a good deal of thought we decided to limit our list of priority areas to the four discussed above.

We close by mentioning three other interrelated areas which have a claim for inclusion in our list. The three areas are 'primary care aides providing domestic and personal care in the home', 'intensive home nursing schemes' and 'the implications of developments in electronics particularly in the spheres of monitoring, data processing and communications for care in the community and in particular community nursing'.

Aides (unqualified staff or sometimes volunteers, with limited (if any) former training for the functions they perform) assist professional staff in providing care in the home in a variety of ways. Such staff with various titles such as care assistants, home aides, home care workers, care attendants and primary care workers, usually employed by social services departments, provide the kind of help to the frail elderly or those acutely or chronically ill at home which in principle a well disposed relative, if available, with the necessary strength, general knowledge and imagination, could equally offer. Night sitting services usually provided by social services constitute a similar kind of lay help at night for those who cannot be left alone but do not necessarily need the constant attendance of professional nursing staff. Nursing auxiliaries working in close support to and under the direction of district nurses represent another relatively common form of lay support for professional staff. The report of the Community Nursing Review (DHSS, 1986) suggests that the work of many nursing auxiliaries 'could be developed into a combination of home help and nursing aide duties', in collaboration with social services departments. UKCC (1986), in its proposals for future education and training for nursing, midwifery and health visiting, recommended that below the level of the registered practitioner (that is to say the equivalent in the new scheme of things of the registered general nurse) there would be aides with relatively limited forms of training particularly suited to the setting in which the aide would work (a period of approximately three months in-service instruction was suggested as a guide). It was suggested that these aides would not be particularly numerous relative to the number of registered practitioners and it was also not envisaged in the long term that there would be a member of nursing staff with intermediate training equivalent to that of the state enrolled nurse.

As UKCC (1986) points out, as the roles of nursing and other health and social services professionals are redefined and developed so it becomes necessary to specify the kind of help via aides etc. which they need to have to perform effectively in these changed roles. This in conjunction with a continuing policy of caring for the ill and frail elderly as far as possible in their own homes rather than in institutions (given the steadily increasing numbers of very elderly in the population) suggests that investigation would be needed into the support of the 'aide' type which professional providers of care in the community will need - the skills required, numbers, forms of training, etc. (See however the work of Challis and Davis referred to on page 250.)

Intensive home nursing schemes represent one means of enabling certain seriously ill or dying patients to be cared for in their own homes - in the nature of things, whatever the cost saving to the health services and benefits to the patients, they make heavy demands on the relatively small force of community nurses (and those in the health and social services supporting them) and possibly on the relatives of the patient receiving this form of care. Studies into intensive nursing schemes of various kinds have been and are being carried out (see e.g. page 194) but it appears to us that there is a continuing need for research into the implications for: community nursing establishments, the wellbeing of community nurses providing such services, and the satisfaction or otherwise of the patients and relatives themselves in relation to various levels of intensity of home nursing activity for any given levels of nursing dependency.

Finally rapid developments in electronics may before long make it much easier for a nurse to continuously monitor the progress of a number of patients in their own homes and such devices as electronic shopping make it easier for housebound clients to conduct their affairs directly with shops, banks, etc. These developments certainly in the long term have implications for the level of staffing required to provide nursing and other caring services to patients in their homes and in due course, but perhaps not immediately, should be the object of research.

Chapter Seven

WHERE DO WE GO FROM HERE?

INTRODUCTION

This book has been concerned with developments in community nursing over the last ten years or so, and research into these developments. In Chapter Two we looked at the background to these developments, in Chapter Three at significant documents and reports affecting community nursing and in Chapter Four at the developments which have taken place. Research undertaken, and priority areas for further research in the field of community nursing, were looked at in Chapters Five and Six.

We conclude in this chapter by suggesting a framework for examining research in community nursing. We consider the strengths and weaknesses of research done so far, how to make the most of research efforts and resources, and end with some thoughts on the whole subject of this book.

A FRAMEWORK FOR EXAMINING RESEARCH INTO DEVELOPMENTS IN COMMUNITY NURSING

We consider here a typical history of the spread of any innovation throughout an organization such as the National Health Service, in relation to the evaluation methods which might be used.

Phase 1. The preliminary phase
In this phase, somebody has a bright idea and it is tried out, quite often by the originator in person. The first report of this initiative would describe the innovation, why it was attempted and show that it can work. Most of the effort goes into the implementation and relatively little into formal appraisal. (There is sometimes an even earlier phase in which someone gets an idea and pub-

lishes an article about the idea but does not try it out - see pages 175-80 for example.)

On becoming aware, from this initial report or by other means, of the innovation in action, others may be attracted to try it out for themselves, perhaps in different circumstances from the originator and some of these will report on their experiences.

Phase 2. The quest for definitive information

By the end of the preliminary phase, if reports sound encouraging, policy makers will be considering what policy should be adopted towards the innovation - should it be generally recommended for introduction, recommended for introduction only in particular circumstances, or, perhaps, discouraged on cost or other grounds? If cost or other implications of its widespread introduction are believed to be considerable, policy makers will be looking around for means of obtaining reliable information on which to base their decision. There are three broad types of enquiry in this context which might provide information of assistance to policy makers at this stage.

a) Surveys of opinion and experience of existing or potential users of the innovation and any existing and/or potential customers of the service with which it is associated may be carried out. These surveys would include both social surveys where a number of persons are questioned using a questionnaire approach, and studies where the 'respondents' were observed or themselves kept records, so as to provide information about relevant aspects of their experiences, for instance of workload, and services provided or received. (See Chapter Five.)

Such surveys would set in context earlier published reports which are often written by enthusiastic supporters of innovations. It is not common to find reports written on innovations which authors judge to be unsuccessful. Surveys would at least indicate whether the innovation was popular with service providers and clients, and maybe why it is so and in which circumstances. How fruitful this line of enquiry would be depends on how widely the innovation has been tried out. It can however be a valuable source of ideas and opinions and experience relating to the innovation and is relatively quick and cheap to execute. (Observational studies are less quick and cheap than those based solely on questionnaires, but we are here assuming that the period of observation is relatively short and widespread, rather than concentrated on a few sites and in depth.) (Some surveys relevant to developments in community nursing are included in the list of surveys included in the references to Chapter Five. For a more general discussion of the use of surveys, see also Cartwright (1983).)

b) Controlled trials. A relatively small series of controlled trials (see page 187) of the innovation could be undertaken. These trials would be in circumstances chosen to be representative of those in which the innovation might be introduced on a wider scale, and ideally representative also of variations of the innovation, so as to identify those which are most appropriate to each of these various circumstances likely to be encountered in widespread adoption of the innovation.

Such trials could incorporate the kind of information gathering approaches in respect of particular examples of the implementation (and control situations) mentioned in (a) above, but would be designed to obtain as objective information as possible on costs and consequences of the innovation in fair, i.e. controlled, comparison with alternatives. The ideal is essentially a randomized controlled trial, possibly multi-centre, of the sort familiar in clinical research. In the nature of things, such trials are relatively long- term propositions and relatively costly to undertake per site of implementation studied and of course difficult to sustain in the midst of the everyday life of working components of the health services such as primary health care teams. Studying a site before and after the introduction of an innovation (i.e. before and after study see, e.g. Bevan et.al. 1979) constitutes an attempt to use the whole site as its own control - how plausible this is depends on whether the site, including its clients and environment, really have remained substantially unchanged apart from the innovation. Sometimes a crossover design is a practical possibility (see page 188).

c) The 'operational research approach'. Operational research techniques, such as simulation, can be used to experiment on 'mathematical' models developed on the basis of existing knowledge about the innovation, alternatives to it and the environment in which it is or might be implemented. Such a model, by varying parameters and inputs and possibly details of its structure can give rapid insight, once the model has been constructed, into some aspects of the behaviour of the innovation under a range of circumstances much wider than could be tried out by trials of type (b) above. Moreover in the idealized world of the mathematical model, it really is possible to use what are in effect randomized controlled trials, whereas in practice something short of this will often have to be settled for when endeavouring to set up a real-life controlled trial of an innovation in primary care. However, findings of the operational research approach would of course need to be corroborated by the use of at least one of the approaches (a) and (b) above.

Information is of course needed as a basis upon which to construct the model in the first place. Constructing a good model is not usually quick or cheap especially in the rather complex socio-technical situation typical of community nursing. However, it is a good way of encapsulating certain kinds of information (including the crucial parameters which characterize a situation and their relative impact upon one another) in a form which could be used to give specific guidance on details for health services staff contemplating introducing the innovation in a particular situation. (Where, as in the case of some recently reported work in the health services, the model can be implemented on commonly available microcomputers (see e.g. O'Keefe and Davies, 1986) it becomes possible for health service staff concerned with the trying out of an innovation to manipulate and interrogate the model themselves directly.) Only one of the studies discussed in this book (B1.1 in the chart on pages 204-9) used such methods, however two other papers which report the use of mathematical models in the context of community nursing are Fernandez et al. (1974), and Hindle (1981).

Phase 3. The monitoring phase

Once an innovation has been widely implemented it will from time to time be worthwhile monitoring its performance to see if it is turning out as predicted or whether changes in circumstances have had some effect desirable or otherwise - also a number of variants in detail to the original innovation may have appeared about which information is lacking. An example of such a study is that carried out by Harrisson et al. (1983), of district nursing outside normal working hours at a time when a large number of districts had implemented one or more of a variety of schemes for providing care of this kind.

The natural investigative tool at the monitoring phase is the survey described under (a) in the methods described for Phase 2. Sometimes a general survey can so to speak monitor a number of features or developments as for example Dunnell and Dobbs (1982). Monitoring, in so far as it identifies problems requiring solutions, or innovative ideas, can set off another cycle of the research process.

STRENGTHS AND WEAKNESSES OF RESEARCH DONE SO FAR

Using the framework among the studies we have examined in Chapter Five, it is clear that the majority are of the Phase 1 kind, namely reports on relatively new ideas recently implemented where the emphasis was on implementation and feasibility rather than on formal evaluation. There was very little evidence of a progression from Phase 1 studies through to Phase 2 type studies, at least of the controlled trial type. There was one example of the use of a mathematical model. (See B1.1 - in references to Chapter Four and chart.) There have been a number of studies of the social survey and activity analysis type, which we list in the references to Chapter Five and which mostly fell into the Phase 3 category (The monitoring phase).

The typical study among those we assessed was made up of a description of the development in its operation and what was done to or for a series of clients receiving a service, often quite a large series and often quite a careful and detailed description. However, because the clients experiencing the development were seldom compared with a control group, comments on consequences were frequently rather speculative.

In only a small minority of studies was there anything which was, or approximated to, a randomized controlled trial (see pages 187-91), though such a trial would have been informative in the case of many, if not most, of the developments studied. About half of these controlled trials involved an element of randomization in the allocation of subjects to 'treatments'. These trials were usually based at one site. (This is not necessarily inappropriate if it is thought that the results obtained on the one site can be generalized to other sites.)

Examination of the studies we evaluated reveals that only very seldom was there evidence of a sustained attack on a subject area by the same group of researchers building on their own and others' previous work (see page 197). Indeed more generally there was not a strong sense in terms of methodology or areas probed of studies systematically building on past work in the way which is arguably the hallmark of successful natural science and which Hicks (1976) and Hockey (1979) advocate.

Hockey (1979) in discussing research into district nursing, stated that 'the development and progession of a long term research programme has advantages over disparate studies'. Hicks (1976) observed

> that one of my disappointments as a layman coming fresh to this and the related fields, is to find so many papers of a "one-off" character and an absence, in the nursing field particularly, of a continuing effort to develop the methodology and the research techniques, to probe in a sustained fashion over a period of time to a better understanding of the nursing activity in the community and to formulate and to test hypotheses by systematic observation.

How serious are these apparent deficiencies - the dearth of properly controlled trials and the lack of evidence of sustained attacks to acquire knowledge of subjects under study? Is the former in fact a consequence of the latter?

In the end it comes down to the question of how much is reliable knowledge about the costs, benefits and other consequences of an innovation worth prior to taking a decision for or against recommending its introduction on a wide scale; and how long is one prepared to wait for such information.

Whilst it may not be easy to give precise answers to such questions there are subject areas where at least with hindsight the costs and other consequences of implementing the right choice from a range of possible innovations are considerable. For example, as Harrisson et al. (1983) showed, out-of-hours nursing schemes can vary a good deal in their running costs with full professionally staffed schemes emerging as very expensive. However, by the time of the start of the fieldwork of this study, most health authorities had taken the step of introducing some kind of out-of-hours nursing service even though they had very little information from evaluative investigations to help them decide which would be most appropriate.

This is not to say that there have been no sustained and comprehensive investigations of an innovation of importance. For example, the series of papers by Ruckley and colleagues (see study B5.1 in the chart, pages 204-9, and references to Chapter Four) on day care after operations for hernia or varicose veins included an examination of medical progress made by patients allocated randomly to one of three diffferent types of aftercare, economic aspects of the various kinds of aftercare, views of community nursing staff and consumer acceptability of day care (consumers being patients and lay caring persons). This added to the body of information provided by Russell et al. (1977) who had undertaken a somewhat similar study at a different site concerned with day case surgery for hernias and haemorrhoids. Important though the question of the pros and cons of day case surgery versus conventional arrangements of care is, it is perhaps no surprise that two of the most methodologically sound and comprehensive studies should have taken place in this area which is somewhat untypical of the problems of primary health care. We say this because, at least from the point in time when the operation took place, the duration over which a given patient needs to be followed in order to obtain information on costs and progress etc. was relatively short. One of the few examples of a sustained attack on a more typical problem of primary care which we encountered was concerned with screening of the elderly and undertaken by Barber and colleagues over a long period (see studies A3.A1, A3.A2, A3.A3 and B3.A1 in the references to Chapter Four) where the fieldwork of the latest and the most sophisticated study in the series alone took some three and a half years to complete. This illustrates the fact that the consequences of the innovation in primary care in terms of the health and happiness of clientele and workers often manifest themselves in a number of individually small ways over a long period of time.

This brings us to the important matter of using suitable means of measuring relevant change in relation to the introduction of an innovation - what changes in the level of resources of various kinds employed are implied by introducing the innovation as compared with the former method of operating and what are the consequences for the various

interested parties: clients, personnel and other
parts of the health and other caring services? In
28 out of the 77 studies we reviewed in Chapter
Five there was no explicit mention of staff or
other resource requirements implied by the innovation though arguably this is one of the easier
aspects of change to measure. In 27 of the studies
outcome in terms of the health and well-being of
patients or impact on any part of the health services was either based on entirely subjective
assessment or (in a few cases) not considered at
all. (See Chapter Five; this is among those studies where we considered that something by way of
outcome, other than that the innovation was feasible, was appropriate.) Some kinds of subjective
data such as the opinions of consumers are important, and indeed in the case of 21 studies of those
assessed in Chapter Five, surveys of consumer opinion were undertaken. However, these were mostly in
studies where data other than the purely subjective
were used to assess outcome (14 out of the 21 consumer studies related to evaluations of this kind).
Clearly an appraisal of the outcome of an innovation which is confined to the impressions of the
professional staff concerned that it has had beneficial effects is of limited use to decision makers
concerned with whether or not to implement the innovation on a wider scale when considered in comp-
etiton with other possible uses of scarce resources.

Good examples of the problems faced and solutions evolved in measuring outcome are to be found
in the work of Carpenter and colleagues (study A4.1
in the references to Chapter Four) in assessing the
impact in terms of lives of babies saved by health
visitor intervention, and in that of Luker (study
A3.B3) in assessing the impact of health visitor
intervention on the lives of elderly clientele.

In reflecting on the problems and possibilities associated with the undertaking of sound and
useful evaluations in primary care settings, it is
a salutory experience to refer to the now classic
'Burlington randomized trial of the nurse practitioner' (Spitzer et al., 1974). To tempt the reader we quote the abstract of the article cited in
full:

> From July 1971 to July 1972, in the large
> suburban Ontario practice of two family phy-
> sicians a randomized control trial was con-
> ducted to assess the effects of substituting
> nurse practitioners for physicians in primary-

care practice. (In fact the fieldwork as a whole extended for a period of several months before the start and a year after the end of the formal controlled trial.) Before and after the trial, the health status of patients who received conventional care from family physicians was compared with the status of those who received care mainly from nurse practitioners. Both groups of patients had a similar mortality experience, and no differences were found in physical functional capacity, social function or emotional function. The quality of care rendered to the two groups seemed similar, as assessed by a quantitative "indicator-condition" approach. Satisfaction was high among both patients and professional personnel. Although cost effective from society's point of view, the new method of primary care was not financially profitable to doctors because of current restrictions on reimbursement for the nurse practitioner services.

No less significant for both researchers and policy makers in this field are Spitzer's sombre reflections (Spitzer, 1984) entitled 'The Nurse Practitioner Revisited: Slow Death of a Good Idea' in which he notes that as far as nurse practitioners were concerned in Canada, 'the programmes, the opportunities for practice, and concrete plans for the future are dead', notwithstanding a formidable array of well designed and executed evaluations which pointed to useful, safe and cost effective roles for nurse practitioners. A coalition of opposing ideas in the form of professional unease about employment opportunities of physicians, remuneration levels of nurse practitioners and general legal difficulties amongst others seem to have emerged triumphant in this sphere.

MAKING THE MOST OF RESEARCH EFFORTS AND RESOURCES - SOME IDEAS

After looking at the strengths and weaknesses of research done so far, some recommendations can be made about future research relating to innovations.

If we take it as given that responsible innovation is to be encouraged on as wide a scale as is compatible with effective day-to-day running of services and overall availability of human and other resources, the relevant policy makers (by which we mean those with some responsibility for deciding whether innovations in their sphere should be explored and/or implemented on a wider scale) can help matters at Phase 1 (the preliminary phase) in the life history of innovation, or earlier, by:

a) creating an environment conducive to sensible innovation; (This is easily said, harder to arrange. Certainly such an environment is one in which ideas are, and are known to be, welcome from any source and one in which care is taken by managers and professional bodies to look for opportunities for their organizations and members respectively in innovations rather than to remain behind the 'Maginot Line' of the status quo).
b) facilitating the rapid and widespread dissemination of bright ideas throughout the service in such a way that they cannot be ignored;
c) ensuring that the training of staff (including in-service training) equips them, technically speaking and emotionally, to innovate and to report effectively and in particular without prejudice about their innovation in action.

Such a policymaker may sometimes need to act as a kind of 'marriage broker' in the sense of matching an idea which seems promising with someone, or with a team of people, in the service willing and able to implement the innovation on a trial basis and to report effectively on what happens. This process is facilitated if the policy maker has a list of these individuals or teams (such as the register of research practices maintained by the Royal College of General Practitioners) and the often quite modest resources needed to enable innovation to be tried out in this preliminary way.
Turning to Phase 2 as we have defined it (the quest for definitive information), it is clear that it is here that the deficiency in the research approach lies. This is the phase where, ideally, policy makers and their professional research advisers should be formulating highly specific sets of questions which need answers by research investigations specifically designed to provide them. This is the kind of research advocated by Rothschild (CPRS 1971). It self-evidently implies a high degree of closeness of contact between the real customer (i.e. the person within the health services who really needs this kind of information in order to take the necessary decisions) and the contractor to hammer out details, and an awareness

of the possibilities and limitations of particular research schemes. Phase 2 type research done properly is expensive and it clearly needs preliminary work to estimate whether this is worth while. Where it is, that is to say where widespread implementation might have major effects in terms of costs and/or benefits, any research design proposed has to be very carefully compared with the norm of a randomized controlled multi-site trial to see how far it is likely to fall short of producing results having the reliability such trials offer.

Where adequate experimentation in real life is not for any reason practicable, at least over the full range of potentially significant conditions and/or variants of the innovation, use of the techniques of operational research, such as simulation, with their foundations in the construction and manipulation of logical models should be considered.

Whatever method is used, assessing the impact of an innovation in terms of its outcome to clients is generally very important and usually difficult to measure. This difficulty is particularly apparent where the likely impact of a change in nursing practice organization is not so much one of life or death or major change in morbidity as in the comfort, relative level of independence in activities of daily living and contentment of clients/patients. In designing Phase 2 type research, the aim of which is in a sense to clinch the argument for or against the spread of an innovation, it is therefore particularly important that customer and contractor hammer out in some detail the measures by which the innovation is to be assessed giving due account to levels of uncertainty inherent in the design of the enquiry agreed upon. It goes without saying that no Phase 2 type enquiry should fail to include a full analysis of the costs of implementing an innovation on a wide scale compared with the existing arrangements to the various interested parties involved - ranging from the patient, up through a particular service and sometimes also to government and society in general (remember that Phase 2 type enquiries are those concerned with important issues). The actual costs of investigation are seldom included in the papers and reports we considered, yet such information is valuable to succeeding generations of research workers and policy makers in formulating a realistic assessment of what it is going to cost to carry out any proposed evaluation.

Where do we go from here?

This brings us to the function of disseminating information on innovations and research which is of course vitally important at the Phase 2 stage if good use is to be made of the quite costly piloting and evaluation of developments which investigation at this stage implies.

Policymakers need to be aware that evaluations have been commissioned - just what the issues at stake are on which they are supposed to provide guidance for decision making and when the necessary information will be available for the decision maker's use. Progress reports both on the date of availability of this information and on what is emerging as the evaluation proceeds (subject always to not prejudicing the fairness of comparisons of the alternatives being examined in the final analysis of the evaluative study by premature and speculative releases of information) keep the evaluation on the policymaker's timetable and agenda. This implies a good rapport and regular exchange of information between customer (or at least 'customer's representative') and research contractor unless as for example in the case of the Care in the Community initiative where a research unit (the Personal Social Services Research Unit of the University of Kent) is commissioned 'to publicize the initiative and to monitor and evaluate the pilot projects' (PSSRU Bulletin, Summer 1986). Various considerations serve to keep the customer (or even the customer's representative in research management) somewhat remote from the contractor (i.e. the body carrying out the evaluation) including the perfectly laudable desire not to be 'breathing down the necks' of research workers when heavily involved in the often exacting business of evaluation. But a sympathetic and informed involvement of the customer in what is happening can do much for the morale of the research workers, offer early warning of any difficulties arising, and pay dividends in offering early insight into the sort of results that seem likely to emerge from the investigation - and in some cases enable changes in direction or emphasis in the evaluation to be negotiated in good time without prejudicing the scientific soundness of the work.

Finally there is the business of disseminating the conclusions of evaluations in a timely and usable fashion to those who need them in order to take decisions (and in some cases to bodies such as community health councils to enable them to make an informed response to decisions taken), and the bus-

Where do we go from here?

iness of maintaining information on 'good practice' both in the delivery of care and the conduct of evaluative research into developments in this sphere. A full discussion of the best ways of carrying out all these information maintenance and dissemination functions lies beyond the scope of this book. However, the Community Nursing Review report (DHSS, 1986) observed:

> It became more and more clear to us, as we visited Districts and studied evidence, that little or no systematic attempt is made to share knowledge and experience of good practice in primary care. We saw uncoordinated effort by hard-pressed health workers who were developing imaginative and effective schemes, believing them to be unique, only to find similar schemes mirrored in other Districts nearby.

Accordingly they recommended that:

> The Government should invite the Health Advisory Service, with its established reputation, credibility and acceptance by the professions, to take on responsibility for identifying and promoting good practice in primary health care.

The Royal Commission on the National Health Service (1979) observed that:

> Health services research is a complex process in which continuity is essential...
> A solution to this critical problem of encouraging systematic research into health care issues would be the establishment of an Institute of Health Services Research... [Among other things] it would encourage the development of a corpus of knowledge and experience in the sphere of health services research, and could help to coordinate the research undertaken by universities and other agencies.

Hunter (1983) examined the matter of promoting innovation in the NHS. He observed that:

> Innovation is necessary to keep pace with, and to anticipate, a rapidly changing

247

> operating environment, including changing needs, resources, demands, and expectations....
> The NHS is not devoid of innovation but it is uneven and ad hoc.

He noted there were several reasons why innovation is difficult to achieve in an organisation such as the National Health Service and proposed that a development agency be instituted to help stimulate innovation and make it work.

> Innovation cannot be left to chance or to the vagaries of the management system - it has to be systematically worked for.

Among the suggestions he made concerning the character of the agency and its working were the following:

> It would act locally with those who make decisions and provide the service, encouraging them to become agents for change... Solutions would not be imposed and the agency would not have automatic right of entry to authorities.
> The agency would not be a monitoring device and it would not try to persuade authorities to comply with national or regional policy priorities or both....
> ...The emphasis would be on promoting innovation through action research and development...
> ...an important priority would be to disseminate good practices derived from the agency's project work and from initiatives by other health authorities.

He also contended that:

> ...the development agency will need some clout to get new developments off the ground.. Pump priming by allocating small amounts of money to launch new initiatives could prove valuable, particularly if, as the present director of the Health Advisory Service claims, the problem does not lie in a shortage of good ideas but in implementing them in diverse working conditions...
> ...A major issue in management is the inherent conflict between hierarchical control systems and imaginative thinking.... A devel-

opment agency could tackle this dilemma: it would not be responsible for achieving innovation in health care but would help to create the conditions for innovation to occur.

A common thread to these recommendations is that some arrangements are needed to build up a store of knowledge about good practice and research activities and to disseminate findings and ideas in a way likely to create the right kind of change in the health services generally and primary care in particular. In this country so far the most favoured solution appears to be to appoint a specific organization such as a research unit, e.g. see page 246, or a body such as the Health Advisory Service to serve this function in respect of a particular set of health problems or service areas. This is in contrast with the Swedish Planning and Rationalization Institute which, as Hunter (1983) mentions, had as its main function:

> to unravel and solve a range of problems confronting the health care sector. Other tasks include disseminating information and supporting research and development work in health care administration.

This brings us back to the kind of problem we faced at the start of this book. Whether it is a matter of producing a one-off account of research and developments in one sector of the health care services or of setting up an ongoing organization to encourage good practice and related research in such a sector, the question is where to draw the boundaries of the field of interest. In either case specialization has its virtues in that it encourages in depth investigation of the limited field chosen. On the other hand if the boundaries are chosen too narrowly or without due regard to the natural linkages between fields of interest, there is a risk that the enterprise will be diminished by missing something of value which lies beyond the boundaries chosen. For example, perhaps inevitably in view of our original research brief, we have concentrated on developments and research in community nursing in the UK as reported in health services literature or by recourse to those working in the NHS, yet it is clear that in contiguous fields such as the social services there are innovations and approaches to research which, while they do not explicitly much involve community nurses, if at all, nonetheless do offer approaches which are applicable and valuable to research and development in community nursing.

As just one example of this we mention the innovation described and evaluated by Challis and Davies (1984). The innovation which related to the care of the frail elderly in the community involved the designation in the case of each elderly person in the experimental (as distinct from the control) group of a responsible social worker

> whose role includes making care at home more effective and achieving more appropriate use of resources by increasing the range of choices open to an elderly person, delaying or obviating the need for unnecessary admission to residential care.

Amongst other things the responsible social worker had control of a decentralized budget.

> This budget could be used upon services or developments necessary to support elderly people in the community and improve their quality of life.

It is not difficult to imagine a similar approach being adopted in community nursing, particularly in the context perhaps of neighbourhood nursing teams as proposed by the Community Nursing Review Team (DHSS, 1986). Challis's and Davies's approach to the evaluation of this innovation with its careful attention to the design of the enquiry and measures of outcome (both in terms of the location of matched cases after one year, quality of life factors, and the outcomes for principal carers, changes in the level of need for various kinds of help and not least differing costs of matched pairs to social services departments, National Health Service and society as a whole) has obvious applications to the study of innovation in some aspects of community nursing.

The point we are making is that given the relative dearth of Phase 2 type evaluations of innovations in community nursing it is a great pity, but all too easy, to miss instructive examples of enquiries in contiguous fields. The construction of data bases relating to research and innovation, with some 'expert' system type capacity to offer an interrogator material which is relevant to the enquiry but not strictly implied by the key words

Where do we go from here?

entered in formulating the request for information,
could help with the problem particularly if such
data bases relating to good practice in various
caring services and fields of interest and research
relating to these were organized via inter-
communicating systems.

AND IN CONCLUSION

In the end it comes down to how best to encourage, channel and support the energies and
enthusiasms of innovators and evaluators so as to
make the best use of these valuable and far from
unlimited resources.
The period since 1974 has for those working
within community nursing been one of considerable
change both in terms of organizational arrangements
and clientele to be served, given demographic and
social changes and government policy to care for
people as far as possible in their own homes and
certainly outside (large) hospitals. For much of
this period, governments have felt it necessary to
limit expenditure on health services to a greater
or lesser degree and certainly in increasingly explicit ways, and this trend persists to the present. In these circumstances, in allocating resources health authorities have been faced with the
dilemma that any savings that may arise from transferring care from hospitals to primary health care
services may only appear in the longer term, yet
the demands made on the latter are more immediate
with corresponding resource implications.
During the period with which we have been concerned the future of the nursing profession generally has been under consideration culminating (see
page 41) in the coming into being of the United
Kingdom Central Council for Nursing, Midwifery and
Health Visiting and the associated national boards
in 1983 as a means of regulating the nursing profession including education and training. At present the UKCC proposals for education and training
directed towards the new professional structure for
those coming within its terms of reference are
being debated. The proposals reflect the increasing professionalization of nursing in terms of
autonomy and accountability within the practitioners' sphere of competence (UKCC, 1986).
Within community nursing, training in order to
practise as a district nursing sister has become
mandatory as it was already for health visitors
since 1981 and a representative steering group has

made recommendations for the training of practice
employed nurses - even though their future has been
the subject of lively debate following the publication in particular of the Community Nursing Review
Team's report (DHSS, 1986). Within health visiting
there has been a sustained and searching examination of the aims and activities of health visiting
and it is our impression that, though problems
remain to be overcome, the profession has emerged
from a period which has not been without its frustrations and difficulties with a greater sense of
assurance as to its actual and potential contribution to health maintenance and care. The report of
the Community Nursing Review Team (DHSS, 1986), the
work of a predominantly non-nursing team, saw a
responsible and challenging role for community nursing and made a number of specific and well worked
out recommendations as to organization and practice, which deserve openminded trial and evaluation. The whole exercise, including the discussions following the publication of a report, has
already done much for the morale of at least health
authority employed community nurses and led to an
increased awareness generally of the contribution
that community nurses might make.

Notwithstanding a variety of frustrations and
problems which those in community nursing have had
to face in the last twelve years, it seems likely
that in the future undertaking of innovations and
participating in their evaluation will for an increasing number of those engaged in this area of
nursing seem a natural and acceptable part of their
work, if pressures of providing care allow.

For the present, it is clear that there have
been many developments in community nursing and
that the research into them has been patchy so that
there are large gaps in certain areas. Whereas
some schemes - for instance utilization of health
visitors in the screening of the elderly - have
been the subject of numerous studies, other areas
have either been rather neglected or studied but
without resolving the issues concerned. It may
seem that a number of the issues arising out of
developments in community nursing which we have
emphasized in our priorities for research in
Chapter Six are 'old chestnuts', for instance the
role of health visitors, or the 'attach versus
patch' question, but these issues will simply not
go away. In the case of the latter issue, for example, over many years there has been both research
(if not so much recently) and much discussion -

however, if anything it seems there is less agreement as to the best way of deploying community nurses in various circumstances than there was a decade ago when Hicks (1976) was writing. On the other hand, the emergence of specialist nurses in any numbers has been a relatively recent phenomenon raising, as we have noted, fresh issues which need study.

Research has been uneven in application for various reasons. Research depends on funding which is often ad hoc, it depends upon research workers being prepared to initiate and carry through the research, upon workers in the area studied - for instance community nurses - collaborating in the research providing records or interviews, and so takes up time and energy which many in the caring professions would be much more naturally inclined to devote to the immediate care of their patients rather than some benefits of an uncertain character in the longer term resulting from research; and research is subject to fashion, since certain topics loom large at one period of time and seem less important at another. Various professional bodies, the health authorities, and the DHSS, may not always agree on what are the most important issues in nursing to be researched. Then there is a problem to start with, where money is limited, in arriving at decisions over research priorities particularly where a longterm programme of research is needed.

Just as research may be patchy and uncoordinated, so is the spread of developments in community nursing. Some developments such as the provision of some kind of night nursing service have become widespread, others, for instance the emergence of the 'nurse practitioner', are rare. Innovations in community nursing depend on ideas being put forward, agreement by health authorities, cooperation of professional bodies and staff and possibly the availability of more resources, in the form of extra staff, equipment or training. As has been mentioned above, certainly there appears to be a lack of dissemination of information concerning schemes as well as about the research which has already been done on schemes, and some possible ways have been mentioned for remedying this. However, any such system by itself is not enough - changes of attitude, for instance on appropriate roles for community nurses, and extra funding, are often needed as well.

Where do we go from here?

The research priorities in community nursing are of course not static. Our list of priorites includes, as we pointed out, both old and new issues. Over the last twelve years or so concerns have changed, as shown in the reports and documents referred to in Chapter Three, and the context of community nursing discussed in Chapter Two has also changed. With the 1980s has come an increased emphasis on cost effectiveness and on the consumer view of community nursing services, areas which were major concerns of the Community Nursing Review Team (DHSS, 1986). At the same time the role of the nurse, for a degree of autonomy and professional independence, has become an issue. And how much should the nurse, perhaps especially the health visitor, aim to change health and indeed other welfare policies, and encourage clients to take matters more into their own hands? The perennial problem is to be aware of longstanding issues which need resolution through further research, and at the same time to be alert to ideas and innovations which arise suddenly and unexpectedly and which also need to be appraised perhaps rapidly.

At the outset of this book we observed that we approached our subject as in some ways outsiders, since we had never practised as health care workers nor were we privy to the (unpublished!) thoughts of policy makers in the field. In two respects however we _are_ insiders. We are present or prospective clients and as such have a vested interest in those who sooner or later will be caring for us or those close to us 'getting things right'. We have, too, spent a good deal of our lives engaged in research into primary health care services and are under no illusions as to the pitfalls and trials that await anyone setting out to undertake work in this sphere, let alone completing investigations that are scientifically sound and decisive. Nothing we have said in this book should be taken to undervalue the considerable achievements of those who have innovated and evaluated these developments in community nursing over the last twelve years.

REFERENCES

CHAPTER ONE: INTRODUCTION

D.H.S.S. (1977) Circular CNO(77)8, Nursing in Prim-
      mary Health Care. Appendix
D.H.S.S. (1981) Primary Health Care Services. Heal-
      lth Visiting, Nursing and Midwifery Staff Sta-
      tistics, England, 30th September 1979. London:
      DHSS Statistics and Research Division
Health Visitors' Association (1981) Health Visiting
      in the 80s. London: HVA
Hicks, D. (1976) Primary Health Care: A Review.
      London: HMSO
Levitt, R. and Wall, A. (1984) The Reorganised Nat-
      ional Health Service. London: Croom Helm
National Health Service (qualification of health
      visitors) regulations (1964) para 2a
Owen, G.M. (1983) Health Visiting. Eastbourne: Bal-
      liere Tindall

CHAPTER TWO: THE CONTEXT IN WHICH DEVELOPMENTS IN
COMMUNITY NURSING HAVE TAKEN PLACE SINCE 1974

Baly, M.E. (1980) Nursing and Social Change. (2nd
      edition) London: Wm. Heinemann Medical Books
Bloomfield, R. and Follis, P. (1974) The Health
      Team in Action. London: BBC Publications
British Medical Association, Board of Science and
      Education (1974) Primary Health Care Teams.
      Report of a Panel. London: BMA
British Medical Association, General Medical Ser-
      vices Committee (1983) General Practice, A
      British Success. London: BMA
Butler, J.R. (1980) How Many Patients? London: Bed-
      ford Square Press
Catchpole, C.P.(1985a) Community computing. British
      Journal of Health Care Computing, 2, 2, 14-15

References

Catchpole, C.P.(1985b) A Survey of the Applications
    of Computers in the Community Health Services.
    Darlington Health Authority in conjunction
    with the Department of Computer Science, Univ-
    ersity of Aston in Birmingham
Clark, J. (1985) The nursing process. Delivering
    the goods. Nursing Times, 81, 2, Community
    Outlook, January, 23, 24, 26-28
College of General Practitioners (1965) Present
    State and Future Needs of General practice.
    Reports from General Practice II. London:
    Council of The College of General Practition-
    ers
D.H.S.S. (1972) Circular 13/72 Aides to Improve
    Efficiency in the Local Health Services - De-
    ployment of Nursing Teams
D.H.S.S. (1975) Staff Training Memorandum STM(75)13
    Nurses Employed Privately by General Medical
    Practitioners (Practice Nurses)
D.H.S.S. (1976) Priorities for Health and Personal
    Social Services in England. A Consultative
    Document. London: HMSO
D.H.S.S. (1977a) Circular CNO(77)8, Nursing in Pri-
    mary Health Care. Appendix
D.H.S.S.(1977b) Priorities in the Health and Social
    Services. The Way Forward. London: HMSO
D.H.S.S. (1980a)Health and Personal Social Services
    Statistics for England, 1978. London: HMSO
D.H.S.S. (1980b) Circular HC(80)8. Health Service
    Development: Structure and Management
D.H.S.S. (1981a) Nursing 1977-80. Report of the
    Chief Nursing Officer of the Department of
    Health and Social Security. London: HMSO
D.H.S.S. (1981b) Care in Action. A Handbook of Pol-
    icies and Priorities for the Health and Per-
    sonal Social Services in England. London: HMSO
D.H.S.S. (1982) Nurse Manpower. Maintaining the
    Balance. London: HMSO
D.H.S.S. (1984a)On The State of the Public Health.
    The annual report of the Chief Medical Officer
    of the Department of Health and Social Secur-
    ity for the year 1983. London: HMSO
D.H.S.S. (1984b)Circular HC(84)10. Health Services
    Development. Reports of the Steering Group on
    Health Services Information: Implementation
    Programme
D.H.S.S. (1985a) General Practice Computing. Eval-
    uating of the Micros for GPs Scheme - Final
    Report. London: HMSO

References

D.H.S.S. (1985b) Health and Personal Social Services Statistics for England, 1985. London:
HMSO

D.H.S.S. (1985c) The Health Service in England,
Annual Report, 1984. London: HMSO

D.H.S.S. (1986) Neighbourhood Nursing - A Focus for
Care. (The Cumberlege Report) London: HMSO

D.H.S.S., Scottish Home and Health Department and
Welsh Office (1969) Report of the Working Party on Management Structure in the Local Authority Nursing Service. (The Mayston Report)
London: HMSO

D.H.S.S., Scottish Home and Health Department and
Welsh Office (1972) Report of the Committee on
Nursing. Cmnd 5115 (The Briggs Report) London:
HMSO

D.H.S.S., Welsh Office, Northern Ireland Office and
Scottish Office (1986) Primary Health Care: An
Agenda for Discussion. Cmnd. 9771 London:HMSO

E.E.C. Council of Ministers (1977) Nursing Directive 77/452. Concerning the Mutual Recognition
of Diplomas, Certificates and Other Evidence
of the Formal Qualifications of Nurses Responsible for General Care, including Measures to
Facilitate the Effective Exercise of the Right
of Establishment and Freedom to Provide Services

E.E.C. Council of Ministers (1977) Nursing Directive 77/453. Concerning the Coordination of
Provisions Laid Down by Law, Regulation or Administrative Action in Respect of the Activities of Nurses Responsible for General Care

Ellis, B. (1985) The nursing process. Making it
work. Nursing Times, 81, 2, Community Outlook,
January, 22-23

Fisher, R.H. (1985) A computer system for the family practitioner service. The British Journal
of Health Care Computing, 1, 4, 10-17

Gilmore, G., Bruce, N., and Hunt, M. (1974) The
Work of the Nursing Team in General Practice.
London: CETHV

Hayes, G.M. (1985) Why don't more GPs use computers
The British Journal of Health Computing, 2, 1,
19,20,23

Health and Social Security Act (1984) c.48

Health Visitors' Association (1975). Health visiting in the 70s. Health Visitor, 48, 322-331

Health Visitors' Association (1981) Health Visiting
in the 80s. London: HVA

Hicks, D. (1976) Primary Health Care: A Review.
London: HMSO

References

Hockey, L. (1983) Primary Care Nursing. Recent Advances in Nursing, 5. Edinburgh: Churchill Livingstone

Hughes, J. and Roberts, J.A. (1981) Nurse Managers' Views of Community Nursing Services. Report to study group B of the North East Thames Regional Health Authority Primary Health Care Working Party. London School of Hygiene and Tropical Medicine, Department of Community Health

Hunt, M. (1974) An Analysis of Factors Influencing Teamwork in General Practice. University of Edinburgh: M.Phil. Thesis

Illich, I. (1976) Limits to Medicine. London: Marion Boyars

Jones, R.V.H. (1986) Working Together, Learning Together. Report of inter-professional learning 1978/85, Exeter Community Training Liaison Group. Occasional Paper No. 33. London: RCGP

London Health Planning Consortium. (1981) Primary Health Care in Inner London. Report of a Study Group. (The Acheson Report) London: DHSS

Marsh, G. and Kaim-Caudle, P. (1976) Team Care in General Practice. London: Croom Helm

Ministry of Health, Consultative Council on medical and Allied Services (1920) Interim Report on the Future Provision of Medical and Allied Services (The Dawson Report) Cmd. 693. London: HMSO

Ministry of Health (1946) National Health Service Bill. Summary of the proposed new service. Cmd. 6761. London: HMSO

Ministry of Health. (1956) An Inquiry into Health Visiting: report of a working party. (The Jameson Report) London: HMSO

Ministry of Health and Scottish Home and Health Department (1966) Report of the Committee on Senior Nursing Staff Structure. (The Salmon Committee) London: HMSO

National Health Service Act (1946) (Applies to England and Wales)

National Health Service, D.H.S.S. (1982) Steering Group on Health Services Information (The Korner Group) A report on the collection and use of information about hospital clinical activity in the NHS. First Report to the Secretary of State. London: HMSO

References

National Health Service, D.H.S.S. (1984) Steering Group on Health Services Information (The Körner Group) A report on the collection and use of information about services for and in the community in the NHS. Fifth Report to the Secretary of State. London: HMSO

National Health Service Management Inquiry (1983) Letter (The Griffiths Report). London: HMSO

Parkinson, J. (1983) Calling the computer. Health and Social Services Journal, 93, 443

Reedy, B.L.E.C. (1978) The New Health Practitioner in America: a comparative study. London: King Edward's Hospital Fund for London

Royal College of Nursing (1976) New Horizons in Clinical Nursing. London: RCN

Royal College of Nursing (1979) Implementing The Nursing Process. London: RCN

Royal College of Nursing (1980) Nurse Prescribers of Oral Contraceptives for the Well Woman. London: RCN

Royal Commission on the National Health Service (1979) Report. Cmnd.7615. London: HMSO

Saddington, N. (1984) Putting Körner into Practice. The Körner Report Five. Nursing Times, 80, 53-55

Scholes, M., Bryant, Y. and Barber, B. (1983) The Impact of Computers on Nursing. An international review (Proceedings of the IFIP-IMIA Workshop on the Impact of Computers in Nursing (1982). Amsterdam, North Holland

Spitzer, W.O., Sackett, D.L., Sibley, J.C., Roberts, R.S., Gent, M., Kergin, D.J., Hackett, B.C., Olynich, A. (1974) The Burlington randomized trial of the nurse practitioner. The New England Journal of Medicine, 290, 251-256

Standing Medical Advisory Committee and the Standing Nursing and Midwifery Advisory Committee (1981). Report of a Joint Working Group on The Primary Health Care Team. (The Harding Report). London: HMSO

Steering Group of the Royal College of Nursing, Council for the Education and Training of Health Visitors, Panel of Assessors for District Nurse Training, Royal College of General Practitioners and British Medical Association - General Medical Services Committee (1984) Training Needs of Practice Nurses. Report of the Steering Group. London: RCN

Sturgeon, C. (1983) Home Computer (computers 1) Nursing Times, 79, 32, 29-30

259

References

United Kingdom Central Council for Nurses, Midwives
    and Health Visitors (1986) Project 2,000. A
    New Preparation for Practice. London: UKCC
World Health Organisation (1978) Alma-Ata 1978.
    Primary Health Care. Geneva: WHO

CHAPTER THREE: SIGNIFICANT DHSS   AND PROFESSIONAL
REPORTS   AND   POLICY STATEMENTS   RELEVANT   TO   THE
DEVELOPMENT OF COMMUNITY NURSING IN THE LAST DECADE

Baly, M.E. (1980) Nursing and Social Change. (2nd.
    edition) London: Wm. Heinemann Medical Books
British Association of Social Workers/Health Visit-
    ors' Association (1982) Joint Statement: The
    Role of the Health Visitor in Child Abuse
British Medical Association, Board of Science and
    Education (1974) Primary Health Care Teams.
    Report of a Panel. London: BMA
Central Health Services Council and the Personal
    Social Services Council (1978) Collaboration
    in Community Care - a Discussion Document. Re-
    port of a working party. London: HMSO
Council for the Education and Training of Health
    Visitors (1967) The Function of the Health
    Visitor. London: CETHV
Council for the Education and Training of Health
    Visitors (1977). An Investigation into the
    Principles of Health Visiting. London: CETHV
Council for the Education and Training of Health
    Visitors (1980) The Investigation Debate - A
    Commentary on an Investigation into the Prin-
    ciples of Health Visiting. London: CETHV
D.H.S.S. (1975) Staff Training Memorandum STM(75)13
    Nurses Employed Privately by General Medical
    Practitioners (Practice Nurses)
D.H.S.S. (1976a)Priorities for Health and Personal
    Social Services in England. A Consultative
    Document. London: HMSO
D.H.S.S. (1976b) Circular HC(76)26. Health Services
    Management: Vaccination and Immunisation: In-
    volvement of Nursing Staff
D.H.S.S. (1977a)Circular HC(77)22. Health Services
    Management: The Extending Role of the Clinical
    Nurse: Legal Implications and Training Re-
    quirements
D.H.S.S. (1977b) Circular CNO(77)9. The Extending
    Role of the Clinical Nurse: Legal Implications
    and Training Requirements
D.H.S.S. (1977c)Circular CNO(77)8, Nursing in Prim-
    ary Primary Health Care. Appendix

References

D.H.S.S. (1977d)Priorities in the Health and Social Services. The Way Forward. London: HMSO

D.H.S.S. (1981) Care in Action. A Handbook of Policies and Priorities for the Health and Personal Social Services in England. London: HMSO

D.H.S.S. (1986) Neighbourhood Nursing - A Focus for Care. (The Cumberlege Report) London: HMSO

D.H.S.S., Department of Education and Science, and Welsh Office (1976) Fit for the Future: The Report of the Committee on Child Health Services. Cmnd. 6684 (The Court Report) London: HMSO

D.H.S.S., Department of Education and Science, Scottish Home and Health Department, Welsh Office (1977) Prevention and Health. Cmnd. 7047. London: HMSO

D.H.S.S., Scottish Home and Health Department and Welsh Office (1972) Report of the Committee on Nursing. Cmnd 5115 (The Briggs Report) London: HMSO

D.H.S.S., Welsh Office (1977) Residential Homes for the Elderly. Arrangements for Health Care. A memorandum of guidance. DHSS and Welsh Office

D.H.S.S., Welsh Office (1978) A Happier Old Age. A discussion document on elderly people in our society. London: HMSO

D.H.S.S., Welsh Office, Northern Ireland Office and Scottish Office (1986) Primary Health Care: An Agenda for Discussion. Cmnd. 9771 London: HMSO

First Report from the Expenditure Committee (1977). Preventive Medicine, Vol. 1, Report. Session 1976-77. HC.169-i. London: HMSO

Health Visitors' Advisory Group of the RCN Society of Primary Health Care Nursing (1984) Further Thinking about Health Visiting. Accountability in Health Visiting - A discussion document. London: RCN

Health Visitors' Association (1975) Health Visiting in the Seventies. Health Visitor, 48, 322-330

Health Visitors' Association (1981) Health Visiting in the 80s. London: HVA

Hicks, D. (1976) Primary Health Care: A Review. London: HMSO

London Health Planning Consortium (1981) Primary Health Care in Inner London. Report of a Study Group (The Acheson Report). London: DHSS

References

MacGuire, J.M. (1977) The Expanded Role of the Nurse (unpublished paper prepared for the Royal Commission on the National Health Service) subsequently published as MacGuire, J.M.(1980) The Expanded Role of the Nurse. King's Fund Project Paper RC3. London: King Edward's Hospital Fund

Ministry of Health (1956) An Inquiry into Health Visiting: Report of a Working Party. (The Jameson Report) London: HMSO

Moore, M.F., Barber, J.H., Robinson, E.T. and Taylor, T.R. (1973) First contact decisions in general practice. Lancet, 1, 817-819

Royal College of General Practitioners (1983) Promoting Prevention. Occasional Paper 22. A discussion document prepared by a Working Party of the Royal College of General Practitioners. London: RCGP

Royal College of Nursing (1976) New Horizons in Clinical Nursing. London: RCN

Royal College of Nursing (1979) The Extended Clinical Role of the Nurse. London: RCN

Royal College of Nursing, Society of Primary Health Care Nursing (1980) Report of a working party on Primary Health Care Nursing - A Team Approach. London: RCN

Royal College of Nursing, Society of Primary Health Care Nursing (1983) Thinking about Health Visiting. London: RCN

Royal College of Nursing (1984) Nurse Alert. A report on the effects of the financial and manpower cuts in the NHS. London: RCN

Royal College of Nursing and the Royal College of General Practitioners (1974) Report of a Joint Working Party on Nursing in General Practice in the Reorganised National Health Service. London: RCN

Royal Commission on the National Health Service (1979) Report. Cmnd. 7615. London: HMSO

Standing Medical Advisory Committee and the Standing Nursing and Midwifery Advisory Committee (1981) Report of a Joint Working Group on The Primary Health Care Team. (The Harding Report). London: HMSO

References

Steering Group of the Royal College of Nursing,
Council for the Education and Training of
Health Visitors, Panel of Assessors for Dis-
trict Nurse Training, Royal College of General
Practitioners and British Medical Association
- General Medical Services Committee (1984)
Training Needs of Practice Nurses. Report of
the Steering Group. London: RCN

Wilson, C.T.(Ed.) (1981) Primary Health Care in
Europe: The Role of the Health Visitor. Report
of a Conference. North East London Polytechnic

CHAPTER FOUR: DEVELOPMENTS IN THE LAST DECADE AND
SOME IDEAS FOR THE FUTURE

CHAPTER FIVE: EVALUATIVE RESEARCH ON DEVELOPMENTS
IN COMMUNITY NURSING PUBLISHED FROM 1974 TO THE
PRESENT (Publications identified by a letter/number
code, e.g. A2.1, are those discussed in Chapter 5
included in the chart, see pages 204-9)

Health visiting

Organizational aspects of health visiting

         Bolton, P. (1981) Contingency plan to meet
             an acute health visitor shortage in
             Thanet, Kent. Health Visitor, 54
             368-369
         Clode, D. (1978) Of primary concern...
             Health and Social Service Journal,
             88, 538-540

A1.1   Dawtrey, E. (1976) The Health Visitor in
             Primary Health Care: a General Study
             of Health Visitors in Two Health Cen-
             tres and a Detailed Survey of their
             Contrasting Work Patterns in One Cen-
             tre. M. Phil. Thesis, Medical Archit-
             ecture Research Unit, The Polytechnic
             of North London, MARU 2/77

A1.2   Gilmore, M., Bruce, N. and Hunt, M. (1974)
             The Work of the Nursing Team in Gen-
             eral Practice. London: CETHV

A1.3   O'Connor, P.J. and Willis, M. (1985) Cler-
             ical help for health visitors. Health
             Visitor, 58, 261-262

A1.4   Poulton, K.R. (1977) Evaluation on Commun-
             ity Nursing Service of Wandsworth and
             East Merton Teaching District. Res-
             earch Report. Wandsworth & East Mer-
             ton Health District

References

A1.5   Walsworth-Bell, J.P. (1979) Patch work. A
        comparative study of the organisation
        of the work of health visitors.
        Health Visitor, 54, 307-310
A1.6   Watts, A. (1985) Health visitor or clerk?
        Health Visitor, 58, 258-259

Health visitors providing services out of
normal hours

        Anon. (1979) Telephone talk. Nursing
            Times, 75, Community Outlook, July,
            199
A2.1   Anon. (1982) Outside office hours (24-hour
            visiting service in Enfield) Health
            and Social Service Journal, 92, 1053-
            1055
A2.2   Beech, C.P. (1981) A new service for par-
            ents with crying babies. Nursing
            Times, 77, 245-246
A2.3   Bogie, A. (1981) A crying baby advisory
            service. Health Visitor, 54, 535-537
A2.1   Haylock, M. (1981) A 24-hours health vis-
            iting service. Health Visitor, 54,
            16-18
A2.4   Metcalf, B., Morris, M., Thompson, A.,
            Unsworth, D. and Hoyle, E. (1981) A
            24-hour health visiting service. Nur-
            sing Times, 77, Community Outlook,
            115-118
        Rawdon Smith, J. (1984) Introduction of
            seven-day health visiting cover in
            Peterborough, Health Visitor, 57, 53-
            54

Health visitors and the elderly

        Dunnell, K. and Dobbs, J. (1982) Nurses
            Working in the Community. Office of
            Population Censuses and Surveys, Soc-
            ial Survey Division. London: HMSO

    a) Health visitors and the screening and sur-
        veillance of the elderly

A3.A1   Barber, J.H. and Wallis, J.B. (1976) Ass-
            essment of the elderly in general
            practice. Journal of the Royal Coll-
            ege of General Practitioners, 26,
            106-114

References

A3.A2   Barber, J.H. and Wallis, J.B. (1982) The effects of a system of geriatric screening and assessment on general practice workload. Health Bulletin, 40, 125-132

A3.A3   Barber, J.H., Wallis, J. and McKeating, E. (1980) A postal screening questionnaire in preventive geriatric care. Journal of the Royal College of General Practitioners, 30, 49-51

A3.A4   Black, S. (1984) Reaching the elderly. Nursing Times, 80, Community Outlook, 266, 268, 269

A3.A5   Curnow, R.N., MacFarlane, S.B.J., Gatherer, A. and Lindars, M.E. (1975) Visiting the elderly. Health and Social Service Journal, 85, 79-80

A3.A6   Currie, G., MacNeill, R.M., Walker, J.G., Barnie, E. and Mudie, E.W. (1974) Medical and social screening of patients aged 70 to 72 by an urban general practice health team. British Medical Journal, 2, 108-111

Freedman, G.R., Charlewood, J.E. and Dodds, P.A. (1978) Screening the aged in general practice. Journal of the Royal College of General Practitioners, 28, 421-425

A3.A7   Gardiner, R. (1975) The identification of the medical and social needs of the elderly in the community. Age and Ageing, 4, 181-187

A3.A8   Heath, P.J. and Fitton, J.M. (1975) Survey of over-80 age group in a GP population based on an urban health centre. Nursing Times, 71, Occasional Papers, 109-112

A3.A9   Joyce, P. (1985) Surveillance of the elderly in the community. Health Visitor, 58, 101-102

A3.A5   Livingston, C. (1974) The Caversham project. Nursing Times. 70, 1591-1593

Neil, M. (1982) It's nice to know that someone cares. Nursing Times, 78, Community Outlook, 243-246

A3.A10   Powell, C. and Crombie, A. (1974) The Kilsyth questionnaire: a method of screening elderly people at home. Age and Ageing, 3, 23-28

References

A3.A11   Smith, A.M., Robertson, R. and Bishop, M.
          (1984) An assessment of the elderly
          patients in a new town general prac-
          tice. Health Bulletin, 42, 234-251

A3.A12   Wightman, F. (1985) The unmet needs of an
          elderly population. Health Visitor,
          58, 99-100

b)   Health visitors and the elderly - liaison
          and 'intervention' schemes

          Day, L. and Mogridge, J. (1981) Health
          visitor who stayed. Health and Social
          Service Journal, 91, 1114-1115

A3.B1   Day, L. (1983) Choices. A Small Study of
          People Aged 75 Years or More Living
          at Home in the London Borough of
          Bromley. Senior Student Report No. 3,
          Health Services Research Unit, Univ-
          ersity of Kent

          Griffiths, A. and Eastwood, H. (1974)
          Psychogeriatric liaison health vis-
          itor. Nursing Times, 70, 152-153

          Halladay, H. (1981) A geriatric team
          within the health visiting service.
          Nursing Times, 77, 1039-1040

A3.B2   Lam, E. (1984) Health visits to the eld-
          erly in general practice. Midwife,
          Health Visitor and Community Nurse,
          20, 326, 328, 330

A3.B3   Luker, K.A. (1981) Health visiting and the
          elderly. Nursing Times, 77, Occas-
          sional Papers 137-140

A3.B3   Luker, K.A. (1982) Evaluating Health Vis-
          iting Practice. London: Royal College
          of Nursing of the United Kingdom

          Thursfield, P.J. (1979) The hospital that
          doesn't say goodbye. Nursing Mirror,
          150, 6, 50-52

A3.B4   Vetter, N.J., Jones, D.A. and Victor, C.R.
          (1984) Effect of health visitors
          working with elderly patients in gen-
          eral practice: a randomised control-
          led trial. British Medical Journal,
          288, 369-372

          Victor, C.R., and Vetter, N.J. (1985) The
          use of the health visiting service by
          the elderly after discharge from hos-
          pital. Health Visitor, 58, 95-96

References

Health visitors and family and child health
care

A4.1   Carpenter, R.G. (1983) Scoring to provide
        risk-related primary health care:
        evaluation and up-dating during use.
        Journal of the Royal Statistical Soc-
        iety, A, 146, 1-32
A4.1   Carpenter, R.G., Gardner, A., Jepson, M.,
        Taylor, E.M., Salvin, A., Sunderland,
        R., Emery, J.L., Pursall, E., Roe, J.
        and the health visitors of Sheffield
        (1983). Prevention of unexpected in-
        fant death: evaluation of the first
        seven years of the Sheffield inter-
        vention programme. Lancet, 1, 723-727
        Dunnell, K. and Dobbs, J. (1982) Nurses
        Working in the Community. Office of
        Population Censuses and Surveys, Soc-
        ial Survey Division. London: HMSO
A4.2   Gillies, E., and Chaudhry, M. (1984) Hea-
        lth education sessions on early ante-
        natal and pre-conceptual health: a
        pilot study. Health Visitor, 57, 81-
        82
A4.3   Harris, J.D.C., Radford, M., Wailoo, M.,
        Carpenter, R.G. and Machin, D. (1982)
        Sudden infant death in Southampton
        and an evaluation of the Sheffield
        scoring system. Journal of Epidem-
        iology and Community Health, 36, 162-
        166
A4.1   Jepson, M.E. (1984) Possibly preventable
        infant deaths: a ten year review.
        Midwife, Health Visitor and Community
        Nurse, 20, 236, 238, 240
        Lawrie, B. (1983) Travelling families in
        East London - adapting health visit-
        ing methods to a minority group,
        Health Visitor, 56, 26-28
        Moulds, V., Hennessy, D., and Crack, P.
        (1983) Innovations by a primary
        health care team: 1. Well-baby clin-
        ics by appointment. Health Visitor,
        56, 295-296
        Moulds, V., Hennessy, D., and Crack, P.
        (1983) Innovations by a primary
        health care team: 2. A postnatal
        group for first-time mothers. Health
        Visitor, 56, 296-297

References

Pahl, J. and Vaile, M. (1986) Health and Health among Travellers. Canterbury: Health Services Research Unit, University of Kent

Pearson, P. (1985) An inner city child health project. Health Visitor, 58, 223-224

Peck, B. (1983) Gypsies - A Sheffield experience. Health Visitor, 56, 365

Phillips, S. (1986) Centre for change. Nursing Times, Community Outlook, 82, (February) 15-17

A4.4   Pritchard, P.F. and Appleton, P.L. (1986) Home based behavioural interventions by a specialist health visitor. Health Visitor, 59, 35-37

Thomas, P. and Sullivan, A. (1983) A mothers' and babies' group in a Family Health Clinic, Health Visitor, 56, 299-300

Tully, M., Miles, S., and Jackson, M. (1983) Child's play. Health Visitor, 56, 341-342

Health visitors and psycho-social problems

Briscoe, M.E. and Lindley, P. (1982) Identification and management of psychosocial problems by health visitors. Health Visitor, 55, 165-169

Clark, J. (1976) The role of the health visitor: a study conducted in Berkshire, England. Journal of Advanced Nursing, 1, 25-36

Clarke, M.G. (1980) Psychiatric liaison with health visitors. Health Trends, 12, 98-100

Drummond, G. (1984) Laughter is better than medicine - a support group for caring relatives. Health Visitor, 57, 201-202

A5.1   Hiskins, G. (1981) How mothers help themselves. Health Visitor, 54, 108-111

A5.1   Hiskins, G. (1982) Personal view. British Medical Journal, 285, 204

A5.2   Mottram, E.M. (1980) The sister's role in group therapy in a general practice. Nursing Times, 76, 253-254

References

Reavley, W. (1981) A joint clinic between health visitors and clinical psychologists. Midwife, Health Visitor and Community Nurse, 17, 337-339

Sarson, P. and Allen, C. (1985) Letter. Health Visitor, 58, 151

Vaughan, J. (1985) Letter. Health Visitor, 58, 151

Webb, A. (1985) Hysterectomy counselling. Health Visitor, 58, 61-62

Health visitors liaising between hospital and community services

A6.1   Ahamed, M. (1978) Follow up of children aged 0-5 years seen in Accident and Emergency Unit, Health Visitor, 51, 84-86

A6.1   Ahamed, M. (1982) A research project, Nursing Times, 78, Community Outlook, 223

A6.2   Firth, D., Chamberlain, M.A., Fligg, H., Wright, J. and Wright, V. (1978) Health visitors in a rehabilitation unit. Nursing Times, 74, 249-250

        Ilett, J. (1984) Liaison health visitor, Nursing Times, 80, 19, 46-49

        Jackson, M.M. (1979) Diabetics at home. Nursing Times, 75, Community Outlook, 123-126

A6.3   Matheson, W.J. and Tillson, H. (1978) The child health visitor. Public Health, 92, 234-236

        Paxton, C.M. (1974) Co-operation and care 1 and 2. Nursing Times, 70, Occasional Papers 113-119

A6.4   Trotter, J.M., Scott, R., Macbeth, F.R., McVie, J.G. and Calman, K.C. (1981) Problems of the oncology outpatient: role of the liaison health visitor. British Medical Journal, 282, 122-124

A6.5   Tuplin, J. (1984) Side by side by district. Nursing Mirror, 159, 23, 33-38

        Wallis, M. (1982) An extended talking service. Nursing Mirror, 155, 10, 24-28

Specialization in health visiting

Baker, J., Grace, J., James, H., and Lindley, B. (1980) A specialized service for handicapped children. Health Visitor, 53, 164-165

References

A7.1   Cunningham, C.C., Aumonier, M.E. and Slop-
        er, P. (1982a) Health visitor support
        for families with Down's syndrome in-
        fants. Child: Care, Health and Devel-
        opment, 8, 1-19
A7.1   Cunningham, C.C., Aumonier, M., and
        Sloper, P. (1982b) Health visitor
        services for families with a Down's
        syndrome infant. Child: Care, Health
        and Development, 8, 311-326
        Dawson, J. (1979) The severely disabled.
        Health Visitor, 52, 262-264
A7.2   Holland, J. (1981) The Lancaster Portage
        Project: a home based service for
        developmentally delayed young chil-
        dren and their families. Health Vis-
        itor, 54, 486-488
A7.3   Houseman, M., Wallace, N., and Wallace, G.
        (1981) The role of the health visitor
        in a psychiatric team. Health Visitor
        54, 354-359
        Murray, J.T. and Baillie, J. (1974) A
        study of the contribution of the hea-
        lth visitor to the support and care
        of terminally ill patients and their
        relatives. Health Bulletin, 32, 250-
        251
        Wilshaw, B. and Aplin, M. (1981) A term-
        inal care and bereavement counselling
        service. Health Visitor, 54, 333 and
        336

Health visitors and screening, surveillance
and assessment (other than for the elderly)

a) Health visitors and the screening of
    infants and children

A8.A1   Berkeley, M.I.K., Dewar, M.E. and Gordon
        Robinson, H. (1984) Preschool devel-
        opmental screening - Testing the
        feasibility of a standard programme.
        Health Bulletin, 42, 297-309
        Connolly, P. (1982) An enquiry into child
        health surveillance procedures under-
        taken by health visitors in England.
        In: Health Visiting: Principles in
        Practice, Chapter 7. London: CETHV

References

A8.A2   Lawrence, W.C.M. and Sklaroff, S.A. (1978)
         Who should carry out developmental
         screening examinations? Health Bull-
         etin, 36, 25-33

A8.A3   Morris, J.B. and Hird, M.D. (1981) A neur-
         odevelopmental infant screening pro-
         gramme undertaken by health visitors
         - preliminary report. Health Bull-
         etin, 39, 236-250

  b)   Health visitors and the screening of
         adults

A8.B1   Austin, W. (1984) A well man clinic in
         practice. Health Visitor, 57, 204

A8.B2   Carroll-Williams, B., and Allen, J. (1984)
         Running a well-man clinic. Nursing
         Times, 80, 37, 34-35
         Figgins, P. (1979) Screen now - benefit
         later. Nursing Mirror, 149, 9, 24-25
         Jones, L.D. (1984) A hypertension clinic,
         Health Visitor, 57, 206-207
         Newell, G. (1984) Working in a well woman
         centre, Health Visitor, 57, 207-208

A8.B3   Rankin, H.W.S., Horn, D.B., Mackay, A.W.
         and Forgan, C.M. (1976) The control
         of coronary heart disease risk fact-
         ors in general practice: a feasib-
         ility study. Health Bulletin, 34, 66-
         72
         Sadler, C. (1985) DIY male maintenance,
         Nursing Mirror, 160, 12, 16-18

District nursing

Organizational aspects of district nursing

B1.1   West Midlands Regional Health Authority,
         Management Services Division (1977)
         Community Nursing Organisation: att-
         achment v. allocation. Salop Area
         Health Authority. West Midlands Reg-
         ional Health Authority, Regional
         Administrator's Department, Birming-
         ham

References

District nurses providing services out of normal hours

Anon. (1981) ...... and at home. Health and Social Service Journal, 91, 861

B2.1   Gillespie, J.V. (1980) Night nursing service in West Fife. Health Bulletin, 38, 187-193

Harrisson, S.P., McCarthy, P., Ruddick-Bracken, H. and Ayton, M. (1983) District Nursing Outside Normal Working Hours in England and Wales. Health Care Research Unit, Department of Sociology and Social Policy, University of Durham

Hornby, A. (1976) 24-hour community nursing - a pilot scheme in the Lancaster area. Nursing Times, 72, 428-429

Jack, M.A. (1976) A home night nursing service, Nursing Times, 72, Occasional papers, 140

B2.2   Martin, M.H. and Ishino, M. (1981) Domiciliary night nursing service: luxury or necessity? British Medical Journal, 282, 883-885

Sims, R. (1981) A community night nursing service in Essex. Nursing Times, 77, Occasional Papers, 133-135

Sims, R. (1982) An 'out-of-hours' nursing service (Pilot scheme in community nursing in Southend) Geriatric Medicine, 12, 7, 50-53

District nurses and the elderly

Anon. (1981) The Polegate Project in East Sussex. On the spot for the elderly. Health and Social Service Journal, 91, 1021-1023

B3.B1   Allibone, A. (1979) Community caring scheme in rural Norfolk. Update, 19, 781-786

B3.B1   Allibone, A. and Coles, R. (1982) A Study of the Cost Effectiveness of a Community Caring Scheme Providing Medical Services for the Patients of a Primary Health Care Team in a Rural Area - England, U.K. Department of Economic and Social Studies, University of East Anglia

References

B3.B1   Allibone, A. and Coles, R. (1984) There's no place like home. Nursing Mirror, 158, 10, 22-23

B3.A1   Barber, J.H. and Wallis, J.B. (1976) An information system on the needs of the elderly. Health Bulletin, 34, 324-330

Central Statistical Office (1985) Social Trends No. 15. London: HMSO

B3.B2   Currie, C.T., Burley, L., Doull, C., Ravetz, C., Smith, R.G. and Williamson, J. (1980) A scheme of augmented home care for the acutely and sub-acutely ill elderly patient: Report on a pilot scheme. Age and Ageing, 9, 173-180

Dunnell, K. and Dobbs, J. (1982) Nurses Working in the Community. Office of Population Censuses and Surveys, Social Survey Division. London: HMSO

B3.B3   Gibbins, F.J., Lee, M., Davison, P.R., O'Sullivan, P., Hutchinson, M., Murphy, D.R. and Ugwu, C.N. (1982) Augmented home nursing as an alternative to hospital care for chronic elderly invalids. British Medical Journal, 284, 330-333

B3.A2   Gooding, H., Williamson, G.H., and Honneyman, F.D. (1982) Developing a preventive care service for the elderly. Health Visitor, 55, 593-600

B3.B4   Opit, L.J. (1977) Domiciliary care for the elderly sick - economy or neglect? British Medical Journal, 1, 30-33

B3.A3   Shaw, S. (1975) The role of the nurse in assessing the health of elderly people. In: Probes for Health. Edited by Gordon McLachlan, Nuffield Provincial Hospitals Trust. London: Oxford University Press

Victor, C.R. and Vetter, N.J. (1984), DNs and the elderly after hospital discharge, Nursing Times, 80, 32, 61-62

B3.A4   Wallace, C.M. (1975) Assessment of the elderly. Nursing Mirror, 140, 9, 54-60

References

Paediatric home nursing

B4.1   Atwell, J.D. (1975) Paediatric day-case
        surgery in Southampton. Nursing
        Times, 71, 841-843
B4.1   Atwell, J.D. and Gow, M.A. (1985)
        Paediatric trained nurse in the
        community: expensive luxury or
        economic necessity? British Medical
        Journal, 291, 227-229
B4.1   Gow, M. and Atwell, J. (1980) The role of
        the children's nurse in the commun-
        ity. Journal of Paediatric Surgery,
        15, 26-30
B4.2   Hally, M., Holohan, A., Hugh Jackson, R.,
        Reedy, B.L.E.C. and Walker, J.H.
        (1977) Paediatric home nursing scheme
        in Gateshead. British Medical Journal
        1, 762-764

Day surgery and early discharge

B5.1   Garraway, W.M., Cuthbertson, C., Fenwick,
        N. Ruckley, C.V. and Prescott, R.J.
        (1978) Consumer acceptability of day
        care after operations for hernia or
        varicose veins. Journal of Epidem-
        iology and Community Health, 32, 219-
        221
        Haines, J.F. and Thompson, H. (1982)
        Short-stay surgery in orthopaedics.
        Health Trends, 14, 73-74
        Hart, C. (1982) Back home to nurse.
        Nursing Mirror, 154, 10, Supplement,
        ii, iv, vi, vii
B5.1   Prescott, R.J., Cuthbertson, C., Fenwick,
        N. Garraway, W.M. and Ruckley, C.V.
        (1978) Economic aspects of day care
        after operations for hernia or var-
        icose veins. Journal of Epidemiology
        and Community Health, 32, 222-225
B5.1   Ruckley, C.V., Cuthbertson, C., Fenwick,
        N., Prescott, R.J. and Garraway, W.M.
        (1978) Day care after operations for
        hernia or varicose veins: a control-
        led trial. British Journal of Surgery
        65, 456-459

References

B5.1   Ruckley, C.V., Garraway, W.M., Cuthbert-
        son, C., Fenwick, N. and Prescott,
        R.J. (1980) The community nurse and
        day surgery. Nursing Times, 76, 255-
        256
B5.2   Russell, I.T., Brendan Devlin, H., Fell,
        M. and Glass, N.J. (1977) Day-case
        surgery for hernias and haemorrhoids.
        Lancet, 1, 844-847
        Shepherd, P. (1976) Early discharge from
        hospital after surgery. Midwife,
        Health Visitor and Community Nurse,
        12, 289-290

District nurses in the treatment room

        Bowling, A. (1981) Delegation to nurses in
        general practice. Journal of the Roy-
        al College of General Practitioners,
        31, 485-490
        Cartwright, A. and Anderson, R. (1981)
        General Practice Revisited. London:
        Tavistock Publications
        Dunnell, K. and Dobbs, J. (1982) Nurses
        Working in the Community. Office of
        Population Censuses and Surveys, Soc-
        ial Survey Division. London: HMSO
        McIntosh, J.B. (1979) Making the best use
        of time. Nursing Mirror, 149, 6, 32-
        33
        Reedy, B.L.E.C., Metcalfe, A.V., de Roum-
        anie, M. and Newell, D.J. (1980) A
        comparison of the activities and
        opinions of attached and employed
        nurses in general practice. Journal
        of the Royal College of General
        Practitioners, 30, 483-489

Intensive Home Nursing

B7.1   Mowat, I.G. and Morgan, R.T.T. (1982)
        Peterborough Hospital at Home scheme.
        British Medical Journal, 284, 641-643
        Peterborough Health Authority (1983) Hos-
        pital at Home, Peterborough: The Pil-
        ot Scheme April 1978-March 1981. Pet-
        erborough: Peterborough Health Auth-
        ority
        Punton, S. (1984) Objective: nursing care.
        Journal of District Nursing, 3, 3,
        20, 22

References

Roper, M. (1983) District nurse plus. Journal of District Nursing, 1, 8, 22,24,38

B7.1   Williams, P. (1985) Hospital at Home. Journal of District Nursing, 4, 2, 4-6

Nursing and related care - joint schemes with social services

Anon. (1981a) Nursing care in local authority residential units... Health and Social Service Journal, 91, 859, 860

Anon. (1981b) Helping hands at home. Health and Social Service Journal, 91, 766-769

Bowling, A. and Bleathman, C. (1982) The Need for Nursing and Other Skilled Care in Local Authority Residential Homes for the Elderly: Overall Findings and Recommendations. Research report No. 5. London: Social Services Department, Hounslow

B9.1   Dexter, M. (1981) Intensive care at home. Health and Social Service Journal, 91, 170-172

B9.3   Lovelock, R. (1981) Caring at home. Health and Social Service Journal, 91, 925-927

Quelch, K. (1981) A choice to stay at home. Health and Social Service Journal, 91, 1336-1338

B9.2   London Borough of Waltham Forest, Social Services Department (1982) An Evaluation of the Home Care Services Based in West Walthamstow. London Borough of Waltham Forest, Social Services Department

Support services for community nurses in the care of the dying

B10.1   Bates, T., Hoy, A.M., Clarke, D.G. and Laird, P.P. (1981) The St. Thomas' Hospital terminal care support team. Lancet, 1, 1201-1202

B10.2   Doyle, D. (1980) Domiciliary terminal care. The Practitioner, 224, 575-582

References

B10.2   Doyle, D. (1982) Domiciliary terminal
         care: demands on statutory services.
         Journal of the Royal College of Gen-
         eral Practitioners, 32, 285-291
         Lunt, B. and Hillier, R. (1981) Terminal
         care: present services and future
         priorities. British Medical Journal,
         283, 595-598
B10.3   Parkes, C.M. (1980) Terminal care: evalua-
         tion of an advisory domiciliary ser-
         vice at St. Christopher's Hospice.
         Postgraduate Medical Journal, 56,
         685-689
         Wells, K. (1980) Social Care for the
         Terminally Ill at Home and the Ber-
         eaved. Report to Kent County Council
         Social Services Committee. Sponsored
         by Kent Voluntary Service Council

Support for district nurses from specialist
and liaison nurses, and from other services

B11.1   Warner, U. (1981) St Mary's W9, Community
         Nursing Liaison Study. Preliminary
         Report. Research Unit, Department of
         Community Medicine, St. Mary's Hos-
         pital, London

Practice nurses

Training courses and associations for
practice nurses

         D.H.S.S. (1977) Circular CNO(77)8.
              Nursing in Primary Health Care.
              Appendix
         Leiper, N.K. (1975) A course for practice
              nurses. Royal College of General
              Practitioners, 25, 537-542
         Mourin, K. (1980) A practice nurses'
              course - content and evaluation.
              Journal of the Royal College of
              General Practitioners, 30, 78-84
         Rankin, I.F.M. (1981) Practice nurses,
              Scotland (Correspondence) Journal of
              the Royal College of General Prac-
              titioners, 31, 506

Reedy, B.L.E.C., Metcalfe, A.V., de Roum-anie, M. and Newell, D.J. (1980) The social and occupational character-istics of attached and employed nur-ses in general practice. Journal of the Royal College of General Practi-tioners, 30, 477-482

Steering Group of the Royal College of Nursing, Council for the Education and Training of Health Visitors, Pan-el of Assessors for District Nurse Training, Royal College of General Practitioners and British Medical Association - General Medical Ser-vices Committee (1984) Training Needs of Practice Nurses. Report of the Steering Group. London: RCN

Wrightson, M. (1975) Practice nurses get together. Nursing Mirror, 140, 1, 41-42

The practice nurse's work in the treatment room

C2.1   Bain, D.J.G. and Haines, A.J. (1974) A treatment room survey in a health centre in a new town. Health Bulletin 32, 111-119

Dunnell, K. and Dobbs, J. (1982) Nurses Working in the Community. Office of Population Censuses and Surveys, Soc-ial Survey Division. London: HMSO

C2.2   Waters, W.H.R., Sandeman, J.M. and Lunn, J.E. (1980) A four-year prospective study of the work of the practice nurse in the treatment room of a South Yorkshire practice. British Medical Journal, 280, 87-89

C2.2   Waters, W.H.R. and Lunn, J.E. (1981) 102,886 treatment-room procedures: implications for nurse training and item-of-service payments. British Medical Journal, 282, 1368-1370

Extensions of the role of the practice nurse

C3.1   Bevan, J., Cunningham, D. and Floyd, C. (1979) Doctors on the Move. Occasion-al Paper No. 7. London: RCGP

References

C3.2   Gibbins, R.L., Saunders, J., Rowlands,
        C.J., Harding-Dempster, J., and
        Cavenagh, A.J.M. (1983) Does home
        monitoring of blood glucose work in
        general practice? British Medical
        Journal, 287, 801-804
C3.3   Marriott, R.G. (1981) Open access to the
        practice nurse. Journal of the Royal
        College of General Practitioners, 31,
        235-238
        Marsh, G.N. (1976) Further nursing care in
        general practice. British Medical
        Journal, 2, 626-627
        Martys, C.R. (1982) Drug treatment in eld-
        erly patients: GP audit. British Med-
        ical Journal, 285, 1623-1624

Extending the role of the nurse

   Nurse practitioners

        Burke-Masters, B.M.A. (1986) The autonom-
        ous nurse practitioner: an answer to
        a chronic problem of primary care.
        Lancet, 1, 1266
        Cohen, P. (1984) Nurse practitioner in
        East London. Nursing Times, 80, 2,
        22-24
        D.H.S.S. (1986) Neighbourhood Nursing - A
        Focus for Care. (The Cumberlege Re-
        port) London: HMSO
        First Report from the Expenditure Commit-
        tee (1977) Preventive Medicine, Vol.
        1. Report. Session 1976/77. HC.169-i.
        London: HMSO
        Gaze, H. (1985) Out in the cold. Nursing
        Times, 81, 9, 18,20
        Reedy, B.L.E.C., Stewart, T.I. and Quick,
        J.B. (1980) Attachment of a physic-
        ian's assistant to an English general
        practice. British Medical Journal,
        281, 664-666
        Stilwell, B. (1981) Role expansion for the
        nurse. Journal of Community Nursing,
        5, 3, 17-18
        Stilwell, B. (1981) Role expansion for the
        nurse....2 Journal of Community Nur-
        sing, 5, 4, 8 and 11
        Stilwell, B. (1982) The nurse practitioner
        at work. 1. Primary care. Nursing
        Times, 78, 1799-1803

References

Stilwell, B. (1984) The nurse in practice, Nursing Mirror, 158, 21, 17-19

Miscellaneous 'extensions' of the nursing role

Anderson, G. (1984) A new kind of caring. Nursing Times, 80, 14, 16-18

D2.1 Barber, J.H., Moore, M.F., Robinson, E.T. and Taylor, T.R. (1976) Urgency and risk in first-contact decisions in general practice. Health Bulletin, 18, 21-29

Barnes, G. (1981) The nurse's contribution to the Medical Research Council's trial for mild hypertension. Nursing Times, 77, 1240-1245

Barnes, G. (1982) A nurse's experience in the MRC's hypertension trial. British Medical Journal, 285, 1625-1627

Bryan, J. (1982) Taking over the pressure. Nursing Mirror, 155, 23, 18-19

Drennan, V. (undated ?1985) Working in a Different Way: a Research Project Examining Community Work Methods and Health Visiting. London: Paddington and North Kensington Health Authority

Drennan, V. (1985) Meeting the need. Nursing Mirror, 161, 15, 49-51

Fullard, E., Fowler, G., and Gray, M. (1984) Facilitating prevention in primary care. British Medical Journal 289, 1585-1587

MacGuire, J.M. (1980) The Expanded Role of the Nurse. King's Fund Project Paper RC3. London: King Edward's Hospital Fund

Marsh, G.N. (1977) 'Curing' minor illness in general practice. British Medical Journal, 2, 1267-1269

D2.2 Martys, C.R. (1982) Monitoring adverse reactions to antiobiotics in general practice. Journal of Epidemiology and Community Health, 36, 224-227

Wilson, D. (1977) Horses for courses at Staines. Journal of Community Nursing 1, 2, 18-19

Whitehead, G. (1982) Hypertension: detection and management by the district nurse. Journal of District Nursing, 1, 5, 9-12

References

Attitudes towards extending the nurse's role

C3.1   Bevan, J., Cunningham, D., and Floyd, C.
         (1979) Doctors on the Move. Occasion-
         al Paper No. 7. London: RCGP
         Bowling, A. (1981a) Delegation in General
         Practice. A Study of Doctors and Nur-
         ses. London and New York: Tavistock
         Publications
         Bowling, A. (1981b) Delegation to nurses
         in general practice. Journal of the
         Royal College of General Practition-
         ers, 31, 485-490
         Bowling, A. (1981c) A nurse practitioner
         in Britain? Chapter 11 In: Redfern,
         S.J. et al (eds) Issues in Nursing.
         Proceedings of the 22nd Annual Con-
         ference of the RCN Research Society
         held at the University of Kent at
         Canterbury. London: RCN
         Bowling, A. (1985) District Health Auth-
         ority policy and the 'extended clin-
         ical role of the nurse' in primary
         health care. Journal of Advanced Nur-
         sing, 10, 443-454
D3.1   Marsh, G. and Kaim-Caudle, P. (1976) Team
         Care in General Practice. London:
         Croom-Helm
         Miller, D.S. and Backett, E.M. (1980) A
         new member of the team? Extending the
         role of the nurse in British primary
         care. Lancet, 2, 358-361

General review of schemes and studies

         Baker, G. and Bevan, J.M. (1983) Develop-
         ments in Community Nursing Within
         Primary Health Care Teams. Part III,
         Report of the survey addressed to
         chief nursing officers. Health Ser-
         vices Research Unit, Report No. 46,
         University of Kent at Canterbury
         Clark, J. (1981) What Do Health Visitors
         Do? A Review of the Research 1960-
         1980. London: The Royal College of
         Nursing of the United Kingdom
         Clarke, L. (1984) Domiciliary Services for
         the Elderly. London: Croom Helm
         De'Ath, E. (1982) A preventive approach to
         family life - the role of the health
         visitor. Health Visitor, 55, 282-284

References

Dowling, S. (1983) Health for a Change: Provision of Preventive Health Care in Pregnancy and Early Childhood. London: Child Poverty Action Group

Ferlie, E. (1982) Sourcebook of Initiatives in the Community Care of the Elderly. Personal Social Services Research Unit, University of Kent at Canterbury

Hockey, L. (Editor) (1983) Primary Care Nursing. London: Churchill Livingstone

Isaacs, B. and Evers, H. (1984) Innovations in the Care of the Elderly. London: Croom Helm

Ideas for future developments

(1983) Editorial: Teams for the year 2000 Journal of the Royal College of General Practitioners, 33, 67-72

Anderson, J. (1983) CAPD - A role of the district nurse? Journal of District Nursing, 1, No. 9, 6,9,10

Baker, G., and Bevan, J. (1983) Developments in Community Nursing Within Primary Health Care Teams. Part II, A review of the literature 1974-1982 Health Services Research Unit, Report No. 46, University of Kent at Canterbury

Chant, A. (1982) 'Stem doctor' melting pot. Health and Social Service Journal, 92, 1462-1464

D.H.S.S. (1986) Neighbourhood Nursing - A Focus for Care (The Cumberlege Report) London: HMSO

D.H.S.S., Department of Education and Science, and Welsh Office (1976) Fit for the Future: The Report of the Committee on Child Health Services. Cmnd 6684 (The Court Report) London: HMSO

Dingwall, R. (1977) What future for health visiting? Evidence to the Royal Commission on the NHS. Nursing Times, 73, 77-79

Faulkner, A. and Maguire, P. (1983) Nursing is more than doing. Journal of District Nursing, 1, No. 10, 9,10,13

References

Field, S., Draper, S., Kerr, M., Hare, M. (1982) A consumer view of the health visiting service. Health Visitor, 55, 299-301

Fry, J. (1984) Relative support. Nursing Mirror, 158, 21, 25-26

Gilmore, G., Bruce, N. and Hunt, M. (1974) The Work of the Nursing Team in General Practice. London: CETHV

Gray A.(1982) Personal correspondence.

Hicks, D. (1976) Primary Health Care: A Review. London: HMSO

Hopkins, A. (1984) Community care: Practical help. Lancet, 1, 1393-1384

Keywood (1978) Attachment scheme or geographical patch? Nursing Mirror, 147, 6, 35

Kratz, C.R. (1982) Community nursing - a prescription for excellence? Nursing Times, 78, 676-682

Kratz, C.R. (1983) Editorial: Which way do we want to go? Nursing Times, Community Outlook, 79, 147

Muir Gray, J.A. (1977) A difficult decade. Nursing Mirror, 145, 6, 36,37

Russell, H. (1975) General nursing practitioner. Nursing Times, 71, 1855-1857

Saint-Yves, I. (1983) The training of paramedics for primary health care. Journal of the Royal Society of Health, 103, 135-137

Slaney, B. (1984) Bring OH nurses in from the cold. Nursing Times, Community Outlook, 80, 283

REFERENCES IN CHAPTER FIVE APART FROM THOSE INCLUDED IN THE CHART (see pages 204-9) AND IDENTIFIED IN THE REFERENCES TO CHAPTER FOUR

General

Baker, G., Bevan, J., McDonnell, L. and Wall, B. (1984) Developments in Community Nursing Within Primary Health Care Teams. Part I, General Review and Summary. Health Services Research Unit, Report No. 46, University of Kent at Canterbury

Cox, D.R. (1958) Planning of Experiments. New York: John Wiley and Sons

References

D.H.S.S., Department of Education and Science and Welsh Office (1976) Fit for the Future: The Report of the Committee on Child Health Services. Cmnd. 6684 (The Court Report) London: HMSO

Hill, A.B. (1984) A Short Text Book of Medical Statistics (Eleventh edition) London: Hodder and Stoughton

List of surveys relating to community nursing published since 1974 inclusive, classified by topic

Each survey listed is marked according to the method of data collection used.

'Q' indicates that questionnaires were used to collect data (either by post or by interview).

'R' indicates that records were used for data. This includes both routine records and statistics as well as specially designed and kept records, such as diaries or forms recording activities, workload etc.

Organization of community nursing

Q, R   Dunnell, K. and Dobbs, J. (1982) Nurses Working in the Community. Office of Population Censuses and Surveys, Social Survey Division. London: HMSO

Q, R   Hindle, T. (1981) Primary Health Care. In: Operational Research Applied to Health Services. Edited by Duncan Boldy, London: Croom Helm

Q   Hughes, J. and Roberts, J.A. (1981) Nurse Managers' Views of Community Nursing Services. Report to study group B of the North East Thames Regional Health Authority Primary Health Care Working Party. London School of Hygiene and Tropical Medicine, Department of Community Health

R   Richardson, I.M. (1974) General practitioners and district nurses. British Journal of Preventive and Social Medicine, 28, 187-190

References

Community nursing services out of normal
working hours

Q, R   Harrisson, S.P., McCarthy, P., Ruddick-
Bracken, H. and Ayton, M. (1983) Dis-
trict Nursing Outside Normal Working
Hours in England and Wales. Health
Care Research Unit, Department of
Sociology and Social Policy, Univer-
sity of Durham

Roles within and for community nursing

    Health visitors

    a)   Health visitors liaising between
        hospital and community services

Q   Paxton, C.M. (1974) Co-operation and care
1 and 2. Nursing Times, 70, Occasion-
al papers 113-119

    b)   Workload and/or activity surveys
        of health visitors

R   Clark, J. (1976) The role of the health
visitor: a study conducted in Berk-
shire, England. Journal of Advanced
Nursing, 1, 25-36
Q, R   Clark, J. (1981) What Do Health Visitors
Do? A Review of the Research 1960-
1980. London: Royal College of Nurs-
ing of the United Kingdom
Q, R   Dunnell, K. and Dobbs, J. (1982) Nurses
Working in the Community. Office of
Population Censuses and Surveys, Social Survey Division. London: HMSO
Q, R   Edwards, J., Luck, M., and Medlam, S.
(1983) Health visitors revisited.
European Journal of Operational Res-
earch, 14, 305-317
Q   Fitton, J. (1981) What health visitors say
they do - a job description approach.
Health Visitor, 54, 159-162
R   Henderson, J. (1978) What do health visitors do? Nursing Mirror, 147, 11, 30-
32
Q, R   Jefferys, M. and Sachs, H. (1983) Rethink-
ing General Practice. London: Tavis-
tock Publications

References

R   McClure, L. (1984) Teamwork, myth or reality: community nurses' experience with general practice attachment. Journal of Epidemiology and Community Health, 38, 68-74

R   Musanandara, T. and Sutton, T. (1984) Health visitors as key workers. Nursing Times, 80, 3, 49

R   Speakman, J. (1984) Measuring the immeasurable. Nursing Times, 80, 22, 56-58

R   Wilkes, J.S. and Nimmo, A.W. (1976) An analysis of work patterns in community nursing. Nursing Times, 70, Occasional papers 13-18

Q, R   Wiseman, J. (1979) Activities and priorities of health visitors 1 and 2. Nursing Times, 75, Occasional papers, 97-104

R   Wiseman, J. (1982) What health visitors do. Nursing Times, 78, Occasional papers 113-116

R   Worrall, J. and Goldstone, L.A. (1982) Management information in health visiting 1 and 2. Nursing Focus, 3, 9, 130-131, 10, 144 and 178-180

  c) Surveys of health visitor opinion

Q   Connolly, P. (1982) An enquiry into child health surveillance procedures undertaken by health visitors in England. Chapter 7. In: Health Visiting, Principles in Practice. London: Council for the Education and Training of Health Visitors

Q   Connolly, P. (1983) The health visitor's contribution. Nursing Times, 79, 38, 30-32

Q   Draper, J., Farmer, S., Field, S. and Thomas, H. (1983) A Study of Health Visiting Practice in the Cambridge Health District Carried Out in 1982/83. Cambridge: Early Parenthood Project

Q   Draper, J., Farmer, S., Field, S., Thomas, H. and Hare, M.J. (1984) The working relationship between the general practitioner and the health visitor. Journal of the Royal College of General Practitioners, 34, 264-268

References

Q   Draper, J., Farmer, S., Field, S., Thomas,
     H. and Hare, M.J. (1984) The working
     relationship between the health vis-
     itor and community midwife. Health
     Visitor, 57, 366-368
Q   Ellis, P. (1982) A case study in method-
     ology. Job satisfaction in health
     visiting - how can it be measured?
     In: Health Visiting. Principles in
     Practice. London: CETHV
Q   Field, S., Draper, J., Thomas, H., Farmer,
     S. and Hare, M.J. (1984) The health
     visitor's view of consumer criti-
     cisms. Health Visitor, 57, 273-275
Q   Thomas, H., Draper, J., Farmer, S., Field,
     S. and Hare, M.J. (1985) The health
     visitor's place of work. Health Vis-
     itor, 58, 125-126
Q   Watson, E. (1986) A mismatch of goals?
     Health Visitor, 59, 75-77
Q   Wiseman, J. (1982) Health visiting: what
     will be its function in the future?
     Nursing Times, 78, Occasional papers,
     49-52
Q   Woods, J., Patten, M. and Reilly, P. (1983)
     Primary care teams and the elderly in
     Northern Ireland. Journal of the Roy-
     al College of General Practitioners,
     33, 693-697

District nurses

a)   Support for district nurses in the
     care of the dying

Q   Lunt, B. and Hillier, R. (1981) Terminal
     care: present services and future
     priorities. British Medical Journal,
     283, 595-598
Q   Wells, K. (1980) Social Care for the Term-
     inally Ill at Home and the Bereaved.
     Report to Kent County Council Social
     Services Committee. Sponsored by Kent
     Voluntary Service Council

References

b) Workload and/or activity surveys
    of district nurses

Q   Battle, S., Moran-Ellis, J. and Salter, B.
        (1985) Spreading the load. Nursing
        Times, 81, Community Outlook, Decem-
        ber 22-23

Q, R   Bleathman, C. and Bowling, A. (1983) Res-
        idential care: if we don't shout now.
        Nursing Times, 79, Community Outlook
        89-90

Q, R   Bowling, A. and Bleathman, C. (1982) The
        Need for Nursing and Other Skilled
        Care in Local Authority Residential
        Homes for the Elderly: Overall Find-
        ings and Recommendations. Research
        Report No 5. London: London Borough
        of Hounslow, Social Services Depart-
        ment

R   Goldstone, L.A. and Worral, J. (1980) The
        problems of variations in work patt-
        erns of district nurses. Nursing
        Times, 76, Occasional papers 45-51

Q, R   Jefferys, M. and Sachs, H. (1983) Rethink-
        ing General Practice. London: Tavis-
        tock Publications

R   Moran-Ellis, J., Battle, S. and Salter, B.
        (1985) Day in the life of a district
        nurse. Nursing Times, Community Out-
        look, 81, November, 8,11

R   McIntosh, J.B. and Richardson, I.M. (1976)
        Work Study of District Nursing Staff.
        Scottish Health Service Studies, No.
        37. Edinburgh: Scottish Home and Hea-
        lth Department

        Salter, B., Battle, S. and Moran-Ellis, J.
        (1986) Where the buck stops. Nursing
        Times, 82, Community Outlook, Jan-
        uary, 19-20

R   Sartain, B. (1977) Community (home) nurse
        workload monitoring. Health Services
        Manpower Review, 3, 4, 21-23

R   Speakman, J. (1984) Measuring the immeas-
        urable. Nursing Times, 80, 22, 56-58

Q, R   Vetter, N.J., Jones, D.A. and Victor, C.R.
        (1984) Projected use in two general
        practices of services by the elderly
        at home. British Medical Journal,
        289, 1193-1195

References

R Watts, D.E. (1976) District nurses in East Birmingham Health District 1 and 2. A study of their work. Nursing Times, 70, Occasional papers 157-164

R Wilkes, J.S. and Nimmo, A.W. (1976) An analysis of work patterns in community nursing. Nursing Times, 70, Occasional papers 13-18

R Wiseman, J. (1980) Hidden messages. Nursing Mirror, 150, 19, 40-41

R Worrall, J. and Goldstone, L.A. (1980) A general study of district nursing in Wigan. Nursing Times, 76, Occasional papers, 21-26

c) Surveys of district nurse opinion

Q, R Bleathman, C. and Bowling A. (1983) Residential care: if we don't shout now. Nursing Times, 79, Community Outlook 89-90

Q, R Bowling, A. and Bleathman, C. (1982) The Need for Nursing and Other Skilled Care in Local Authority Residential Homes for the Elderly: Overall Findings and Recommendations. Research Report no. 5. London: London Borough of Hounslow, Social Services Department

Q, R Dunnell, K. and Dobbs, J. (1982) Nurses Working in the Community. Office of Population Censuses and Surveys, Social Survey Division. London: HMSO

Q Poulton, K.R. (1981) Perceptions of Wants and Needs by Nurses and their Patients. Wandsworth and East Merton Teaching District

Q Woods, J., Patten, M., and Reilly, P. (1983) Primary care teams and the elderly in Northern Ireland. Journal of the Royal College of General Practitioners, 33, 693-697

Practice nurses

Q, R Dunnell, K. and Dobbs, J. (1982) Nurses Working in the Community. Office of Population Censuses and Surveys, Social Survey Division. London: HMSO

References

Q   Reedy, B.L.E.C., Philips, P.R., Newell, D.J. (1976) Nurses and nursing in primary medical care in England. British Medical Journal, 2, 1304-1306

Q   Reedy, B.L.E.C., Metcalfe, A.V., de Roumanie, M. and Newell, D.J. (1980) The social and occupational characteristics of attached and employed nurses in general practice. Journal of the Royal College of General Practitioners, 30, 477-482

Q   Reedy, B.L.E.C., Metcalfe, A.V., de Roumanie, M. and Newell, D.J. (1980) A comparison of the activities and opinions of attached and employed nurses in general practice. Journal of Royal College of General Practitioners, 30, 483-489

Q   Sanders, D.J., Stone, V., Fowler, G. and Marzillier, J. (1986) Practice nurses and antismoking education. British Medical Journal, 292, 381-383

Other

a) Surveys of views on extending the role of the nurse

Q   Bowling, A. (1981) Delegation to nurses in general practice. Journal of the Royal College of General Practitioners, 31, 485-490

Q   Bowling, A. (1981) Delegation in General Practice. A Study of Doctors and Nurses. London and New York: Tavistock Publications

Q   Bowling, A. (1985) Doctors and nurses: delegation and substitution. In: Health Care UK - 1985, ed. by Harrison, A. and Gretton, J. London: Chartered Institute of Public Finance and Accountancy

Q   Miller, D.S. and Backett, E.M. (1980) A new member of the team? Extending the role of the nurse in British primary care. The Lancet, 2, 358-361

References

b) **District nurses, practice nurses, and the treatment room**
    (see also papers by Reedy et al. listed on on page 289-90).

Q   Cartwright, A. and Anderson, R. (1981)
        General Practice Revisited. London:
        Tavistock Publications
R   Nimmo, A.W. (1978) Treatment room work: an
        analysis 1 and 2. Nursing Times, 74,
        Occasional papers, 109-116

The consumer viewpoint and experience

Q   Biswas, B. and Sands, C. (1984) Mothers'
        reasons for attending a child health
        clinic. Health Visitor, 57, 41-42
Q   Bolton, P. (1984) A survey of child health
        clinics in Thanet, Kent. Health Vis-
        itor, 57, 42-43
Q   Cartwright, A. and Anderson, R. (1981)
        General Practice Revisited, London:
        Tavistock Publications
Q   Cartwright, A. and Anderson, R. (1979)
        Patients and their Doctors. Occa-
        sional Paper No. 8. London: RCGP
Q   Clark, J. (1984) Mothers' perceptions of
        health visiting. Health Visitor, 57,
        265-268
Q   Field, S., Draper, J., Kerr, M. and Hare,
        M. (1982) A consumer view of the hea-
        lth visiting service. Health Visitor,
        55, 299-301
Q   Foxman, R., Moss, P., Bolland, G.and Owen,
        C. (1982) A consumer view of the hea-
        lth visitor at six weeks post-partum.
        Health Visitor, 55, 302-308
Q   Mayall, B. and Grossmith, C. (1985) Caring
        for the health of young children - 3.
        The health visitor and the provision
        of services. Health Visitor, 58, 349-
        352
Q   Moss, P., Bolland, G., Foxman, R. and
        Owen, C. (1986) The first six months
        after birth: mothers' views of health
        visitors. Health Visitor, 59, 71-74
Q   Orr, J. (1980) Health Visiting in Focus. A
        consumer's view of health visiting in
        Northern Ireland. London: Royal Coll-
        ege of Nursing of the United Kingdom

References

Q   Poulton, K.R. (1981) Perceptions of Wants and Needs by Nurses and their Patients. Wandsworth and East Merton Teaching District

Q, R   Robinson, J. (1982) An Evaluation of Health Visiting. London: Council for the Education and Training of Health Visitors

Q   Sefi, S. and Macfarlane, A. (1985) Child health clinics: why mothers attend. Health Visitor, 58, 129-130

Q   Simms, M. and Smith, C. (1984) Teenage mothers; some views on health visitors. Health Visitor, 57, 269-270

Q   Watson, E. (1982) Problems of the health visitor in the inner city. Health Visitor, 55, 574-576

Q   Watson, E. (1984) Health of infants and use of health services by mothers of different ethnic groups in East London. Community Medicine, 6, 117-135

Q   Watson, E. (1986) A mismatch of goals? Health Visitor, 59, 75-77

Other

Staffing levels, manpower

R   Abel, P.M., Farmer, P.J., Hunter, M.H.S. and Shipp, P.J. (1976) Nursing manpower 1 and 2. A sound statistical base for policy making. Nursing Times, 70, Occasional papers 1-7

Q, R   Burrell-Davis, L. and Williams, W.M. (1984) Health visitor manpower survey 1979-1981. Health Visitor, 57, 9-14

R   Down, J. and Snaith, A.H. (1975) The deployment of home nurses. British Journal of Preventive and Social Medicine, 29, 53-57

R   Jones, R. (1981) A measure of support. Nursing Mirror, 153, 13, 30-31

R   Harris, E. (1977) District nurses: how many in AD 2,000? Nursing Mirror, 145, 6, 35-36

Q, R   Hughes, J., Stockton, P., Roberts, J.A. and Logan, R.F.L. (1979) Nurses in the community: a manpower study. Journal of Epidemiology and Community Health, 33, 262-269

References

R   Whitaker, M.S.R. (1977) A district nurse
         work analysis: a method of measuring
         work and staff levels. Nursing Times,
         73, 97-100

Team development

Q   Gilmore, M., Bruce, N. and Hunt, M. (1974)
         The Work of the Nursing Team in Gen-
         eral Practice. London: Council for
         the Education and Training of Health
         Visitors
Q   Strang, J.R., Caine, N. and Acheson, R.M.
         (1983) Team care of elderly patients
         in general practice. British Medical
         Journal, 286, 851-854
Q   Tatara, K., Sasai, Y., Ogawa, S., Cho, T.
         and Asakura, S. and Bevan, J.M.
         (1982) Co-operation between general
         practitioners and community nurses
         based at health centres and other
         types of premises in the United King-
         dom as seen through the eyes of Jap-
         anese doctors, 1979, Public Health,
         96, 79-85

Views of chief nursing officers

Q   Baker, G. and Bevan, J.M. (1983) Develop-
         ments in Community Nursing Within
         Primary Health Care Teams, Part III
         Report of the survey addressed to
         chief nursing officers. Health Ser-
         vices Research Unit, Report No. 46,
         University of Kent at Canterbury
Q   Bowling, A. (1985) District health author-
         ity policy and the 'extended clinical
         role of the nurse' in primary health
         care. Journal of Advanced Nursing,
         10, 443-454

Care for increased numbers of elderly

Q   Ferlie, E. (1982) Sourcebook of Innova-
         tions in the Community Care of the
         Elderly, Personal Social Services
         Research Unit, University of Kent at
         Canterbury

References

CHAPTER SIX: IDENTIFYING THE PRIORITIES FOR
FUTURE RESEARCH

(1982) Editorial: The need for a national inquiry
    into the proper role and functions of health
    visitors and school nurses. Health Visitor,
    55, 445
Clark, J. (1981) What Do Health Visitors Do? A
    Review of the Research 1960-1980. London:
    Royal College of Nursing
Connolly, P. (1982) An enquiry into child health
    surveillance procedures undertaken by health
    visitors in England. In: Health Visiting:
    Principles in Practice, Chapter 7, London:
    CETHV
D.H.S.S. (1986) Neighbourhood Nursing - A Focus
    for Care. (The Cumberlege Report) London: HMSO
D.H.S.S., Welsh Office, Northern Ireland Office and
    Scottish Office (1986) Primary Health Care: An
    Agenda for Discussion. Cmnd. 9771. London:
    HMSO
Dawtrey, E. (1976) The Health Visitor in Primary
    Health Care: a General Study of Health Visit-
    ors in Two Health Centres and a Detailed Sur-
    vey of their Contrasting Work Patterns in One
    Centre. M.Phil. Thesis, Medical Arthitecture
    Research Unit, The Polytechnic of North Lon-
    don, MARU 2/77
Dingwall, R. and Watson, P. (1980) Pausing before a
    rush to change. Health and Social Service
    Journal, 90, 749-750
Dunnell, K. and Dobbs, J. (1982) Nurses Working in
    the Community. Office of Population Censuses
    and Surveys, Social Survey Division. London:
    HMSO
Goodwin, S. (1982) A cure for all ills? Nursing
    Mirror, 154, 22, 20-22
Harrisson, S.P., McCarthy, P., Ruddick-Bracken, H.
    and Ayton, M. (1983) District Nursing Outside
    Normal Working Hours in England and Wales.
    University of Durham, Health Care Research
    Unit, Department of Sociology and Social Pol-
    icy
Health Visitors' Association (1981) Health Visiting
    in the 80s. London: HVA
Hicks, D. (1976) Primary Health Care: A Review.
    London: HMSO
Hockey, L. (1984) Is the practice nurse a good
    idea? Journal of the Royal College of General
    Practitioners, 34, 102-103

References

London Health Planning Consortium (1981) Primary Health Care in Inner London. Report of a Study Group. (The Acheson Report) London: DHSS

Martin, M.H. and Ishino, M. (1981) Domiciliary night nursing service: luxury or necessity? British Medical Journal, 282, 883-885

Ministry of Health (1956) An Inquiry into Health Visiting: Report of a Working Party (The Jameson Report) London: HMSO

National Health Service Management Inquiry (1983) Letter (The Griffiths Report) London: HMSO

Poulton, K.R. (1977) Evaluation on Community Nursing Service of Wandsworth and East Merton Teaching District. Research Report. Wandsworth and East Merton Health District

Royal College of Nursing, Society of Primary Health Care Nursing (1983) Thinking About Health Visiting. London: RCN

Standing Medical Advisory Committee and the Standing Nursing and Midwifery Advisory Committee (1981) Report of a Joint Working Group on The Primary Health Care Team. (The Harding Report) London: HMSO

United Kingdom Central Council for Nurses, Midwives and Health Visitors (1986) Project 2000. A New Preparation for Practice. London: UKCC

Walsworth Bell, J.P. (1979) Patch work. A comparative study of the organization of the work of health visitors. Health Visitor, 54, 307-310

West Midlands Regional Health Authority, Management Services Division (1977) Community Nursing Organisation: Attachment v. Allocation. Salop Area Health Authority. West Midlands Regional Health Authority, Regional Administrator's Department, Birmingham

CHAPTER SEVEN: WHERE DO WE GO FROM HERE?

Bevan, J., Cunningham, D. and Floyd, C. (1979) Doctors on the Move. Occasional Paper No. 7. London: RCGP

Cartwright, A. (1983) Health Surveys in Practice and in Potential. London: King Edward's Hospital Fund for London

Central Policy Review Staff (1971) The Organisation and Management of Government Research and Development. (The Rothschild Report) Cmnd. 4814. London: HMSO

References

Challis, D. and Davies, B. (1984) Home care of the frail elderly: matching resources to needs. Home Health Care Services Quarterly, 3/4, Fall, 89-108

D.H.S.S. (1986) Neighbourhood Nursing - A Focus for Care. (The Cumberlege Report) London: HMSO

Dunnell, K. and Dobbs, J. (1982) Nurses Working in the Community. Office of Population Censuses and Surveys, Social Survey Division. London: HMSO

Fernandez, A. Gregory, G., Hindle, A. and Lee, A.C. (1974) A model for community nursing in a rural county. Operational Research Quarterly, 25, 231-239

Harrisson, S.P., McCarthy, P., Ruddick-Bracken, H. and Ayton, M. (1983) District Nursing Outside Normal Working Hours in England and Wales. Health Care Research Unit, Department of Sociology and Social Policy, University of Durham

Hicks, D. (1976) Primary Health Care: A Review. London: HMSO

Hindle, T. (1981) Primary Health Care. In: Operational Research Applied to Health Services. Edited by Duncan Boldy, London: Croom Helm

Hockey, L. (1979) A Study of District Nursing. PhD Thesis, City University

Hunter, D.J. (1983) Promoting innovation in the NHS. British Medical Journal, 286, 736-738

O'Keefe, R., and Davies, R. (1986) A microcomputer system for simulation modelling. European Journal of Operational Research, 24, 23-29

Royal Commission on the National Health Service (1979) Report, Cmnd. 7615. London: HMSO

Russell, I.T., Brendan Devlin, H., Fell, M. and Glass, N.J. (1977) Day-case surgery for hernias and haemorrhoids. Lancet, 1, 844-847

Spitzer, W.O., Sackett, D.L., Sibley, J.C., Roberts, R.S., Gent, M., Kergin, D.J., Hackett, B.A. and Olynich, A. (1974) The Burlington randomized trial of the nurse practitioner. The New England Journal of Medicine, 290, 251-256

Spitzer, M.D. (1984) The nurse practitioner revisited. Slow death of a good idea. The New England Journal of Medicine, 310, 1049-1051

United Kingdom Central Council for Nurses, Midwives and Health Visitors (1986) Project 2000. A New Preparation for Practice. London: UKCC